8-16-07

A GUIDE TO GETTING THE BEST HEALTH CARE FOR YOUR CHILD

Roy Benaroch, M.D.

The Praeger Series on Contemporary Health and Living
Julie Silver, Series Editor

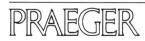

Westport, Connecticut
London

Library of Congress Cataloging-in-Publication Data

Benaroch, Roy.
   A guide to getting the best health care for your child / Roy Benaroch.
      p. cm.—(The Praeger series on contemporary health and living, ISSN 1932–8079)
   Includes bibliographical references and index.
   ISBN-10: 0–275–99346–9–ISBN-13: 978–0–275–99346–7 (alk. paper)
      1. Children—Health and hygiene.   2. Child health services.
3. Parent and child.   I. Title.
   RJ102.B44   2007
   618.92–dc22   2006028559

British Library Cataloguing in Publication Data is available.

Library of Congress Catalog Card Number: 2006028559
ISBN-10: 0–275–99346–9
ISBN-13: 978–0–275–99346–7
ISSN: 1932–8079

First published in 2007

Praeger Publishers, 88 Post Road West, Westport, CT 06881
An imprint of Greenwood Publishing Group, Inc.
www.praeger.com

Printed in the United States of America

∞™

The paper used in this book complies with the
Permanent Paper Standard issued by the National
Information Standards Organization (Z39.48–1984).

10 9 8 7 6 5 4 3 2 1

This book is for general information only. No book can ever substitute for the judgment of a
medical professional. If you have worries or concerns, contact your doctor.

The names and many details of individuals discussed in this book have been changed to protect the
patients' identities. Some of the stories are composites of patient interactions created for illustrative
purposes.

For Jodi

CONTENTS

SERIES FOREWORD

Over the past hundred years, there have been incredible medical break-throughs that have prevented or cured illness in billions of people and helped many more improve their health while living with chronic conditions. A few of the most important twentieth–century discoveries include antibiotics, organ transplants, and vaccines. The twenty-first century has already heralded important new treatments including such things as a vaccine to prevent human papillomavirus from infecting and potentially leading to cervical cancer in women. Polio is on the verge of being eradicated worldwide, making it only the second infectious disease behind smallpox to ever be erased as a human health threat.

In this series, experts from many disciplines share with readers important and updated medical knowledge. All aspects of health are considered including subjects that are disease-specific and preventive medical care. Disseminating this information will help individuals to improve their health as well as researchers to determine where there are gaps in our current knowledge and policy-makers to assess the most pressing needs in health care.

Series Editor Julie Silver, M.D.
Assistant Professor
Harvard Medical School
Department of Physical Medicine and Rehabiliation

PREFACE

Secrets.
Everyone's got them.

Every profession has its secrets, known only to true insiders. Only the chef knows the secret ingredient in your favorite restaurant's lasagna. After the mechanic has poked under a car's hood, very few of us know how to argue with the $600 bill. There's a secret way to get the best concert tickets, and a secret way to know which loaf of bread has been on the shelf the longest.

Fortunately, most of these secrets really don't matter. You might overpay the mechanic, or you might not be able to make the best lasagna at home. But not knowing the inside information about these businesses shouldn't worry you. It's nice to know that the secret of buying the freshest bread at the supermarket is in the color of the twist ties (the color usually correlates in alphabetical order with the days of the week), but it really isn't important.

What about another profession, one you depend on for the health of your children? Could pediatricians have their own secrets and their own insider information?

You bet we do.

Medicine has always had its secrets. Our language is inscrutable, our handwriting is deplorable, and even if you could read it much of what we write is in Latin abbreviations. Each medical discipline has its own conventions and shorthand, and doctors each have their own favorite collections of cryptic jargon and codified notations. Every medication is called by at least two different names, and many diseases have multiple synonyms that go in and out of style. Likewise, the business side of medicine would probably make no sense to an outsider. Few people actually pay our posted prices, and many of us could make more money by seeing some of our patients *less* frequently.

You may think that your pediatrician will always have your best interests at heart. I sincerely believe that most pediatricians really do. But you should know that there is more than experience and medical judgment that goes into your physician's recommendations. There are ubiquitous sales people pushing the latest wonderdrug, and there are insurance companies watching how often we refer patients to specialists. There is an ever-present specter of malpractice litigation. There are also fears: fear of making a mistake, fear of disappointing a family, fear of losing business, and fear of losing a patient. Many issues lurk beneath the surface, and even the most well-meaning pediatricians may not realize just how much these influence their medical advice.

This book will help parents understand the practice of health care for children from an insider's point of view. You'll discover tips on how to find the best pediatricians, and how to make sure that they've kept their knowledge sharp. You'll find out how to get the most out of encounters with your doctors, whether they're in person or on the phone. You'll see the best ways to use your doctor's office: how to minimize waits, get free samples, and have your child's camp forms filled out quickly in an emergency. The real inside story on medicines, labs, tests, and alternative therapies will surprise you, but you need to know the facts to help make the best decisions for your family. Dealing with your children's health means dealing with insurance, and you'll discover the best ways not only to choose insurance, but also to get the most value out of your policy. You'll learn how to help your child through a trip to the emergency room, and how to protect your children from harmful medical mistakes.

The practical and usable advice of a pediatric insider can help you get the best health care for your children. You can certainly get *good* medical care without knowing the inside story. With the knowledge of *A Guide to Getting the Best Health Care for Your Child*, you'll be able to get medical care that is better.

Everyone has secrets, and it's time for this pediatric insider to tell you his.

ACKNOWLEDGMENTS

I began writing this book several years ago, though I didn't know it then. With the encouragement and support of many people, what began as my own personal ruminations and transcribed mutterings became what I hope is a genuinely useful resource for parents.

Thanks to my sweetie, my editor, and my love, Jodi. Keeping the kids quiet and distracted so I could write during our "spare time" was no small feat. My heart is yours.

Thanks to Hannah, Daniel, and Sophie for helping me laugh and enjoy life.

Thanks to Debbie Carvalko and Julie Silver with Praeger Publishing for their enthusiasm for my very first book. I tossed a cool idea onto their desk, and they let me get away with it.

Thanks to my partners Jose and Patty de Urioste. They have taught me a tremendous amount about pediatrics and business, and I could not have gotten so far without their friendship and good judgment.

Thanks to my Mom and Dad for their love and for putting education first. As Dad said, I could do anything I wanted to—after medical school! I know he would be proud.

Thanks to Lee, Gilly, Cindy, Terri, Traci, Jennifer, and Bonnie for early reads, ideas, and confidence.

My biggest thanks go to my patients, who've taught me—more than anyone else—what I really need to know. I am honored by your trust. Though I cannot possibly list even a fraction of the many families whose faces and lessons I remember, there are a few that I would like to thank personally and by name. I've listed just the initials of your kids; you know who you are. Special thanks for what you've taught me: PA, CA, DA, OA, WB, CB, BB, MC, CC, AC, KF, KG, BL, DM, CM, MM, ZS, PS, and DV.

1

FIND YOUR DREAM PEDIATRICIAN

A few years ago I was examining a very curious eight-year-old boy. I try to answer every question, especially the ones posed by the kids, but I was having trouble keeping up with his rapid fire interrogation. Mom tried to help me out by asking an easy one, "How do you become a pediatrician?" My patient jumped in with the answer before I could open my mouth. "First, you get a teeeeeeeny stethoscope."

What is a pediatrician? We're physicians trained exclusively to take care of kids, from premature babies through college students. We're the ones who don't mind the crying, the whining, and the midnight phone calls. We chose to do this, and it is the best job in the world.

A pediatrician is the most qualified person to help your family with children's health care issues. To choose the best one, you'll want to know the inside story on the doctors devoted to the health of children. Why did we choose pediatrics, and how are we trained? You'll also need to know the practical clues and tips that can help you find the best office with the best pediatrician for your child.

BECOMING A PEDIATRICIAN

I remember a surprised medical school dean asking me why I was choosing pediatrics. After all, pediatricians are among the lowest paid doctors, and we rate low on the pecking order among other physicians. If all of medicine were one big dog, the pediatric department would be the tail: we're cute, we wag, and we're nice to have around—after all, the dog would look a little peculiar without a tail. But to the overall medical profession, we're really not considered a specialty to be taken seriously.

Not having to be too serious is one reason many of us chose to become pediatricians. We like talking with children and making babies laugh. We enjoy our role as teachers, helping both parents and children learn the skills they need. Our patients are moving targets: babies become toddlers who become children and then teens. Every stage has its own challenges and rewards for parents and pediatricians both. Our goal is to watch every baby in our practice grow into a well-adjusted and healthy teenager. In short, pediatricians choose their field for the joy and rewards of helping children grow.

Though we may seem less intense than our adult medicine colleagues, our pediatric training is rigorous and extensive. Even those of us who sometimes act particularly silly consider children's health a very serious matter. A pediatrician's education starts with a four year college degree followed by four years of medical school, then three years of pediatric residency training. To call yourself a pediatrician, you have to complete the required training at an accredited program, and pass a national board exam. Pediatricians currently completing their training have to requalify every seven years in a process that includes continuing education classes, proof of professional competence, and further board examinations. American pediatricians who are fully qualified should have the letters "FAAP" after the "MD," as in Roy Benaroch, MD, FAAP. This means Fellow, American Academy of Pediatrics.

Pediatric residency training covers both inpatient and outpatient medicine, from the care of the sickest premature babies in the neonatal intensive care unit to the management of toilet training problems; from the care of teenagers with gunshot wounds to the counseling of first time moms. Teaching in residency is through both lectures and practical experience. Many of the most memorable lessons occur at unexpected times: a nurse shows you the best way to swaddle and calm a newborn, a teenager reveals that school makes her stomach hurt, or an energetic emergency room physician explains how to splint an ankle at 3 am. It's a whirlwind of three years, and for the best pediatricians it is only the beginning of learning how to take care of children.

The Words of Medical Education

Medical school: A four-year postgraduate program that confers an MD (Doctor of Medicine) or DO (Doctor of Osteopathy) degree. Traditionally, the first two years are "book learning" and the second two years are a series of clinical "clerkships" where medical students spend a month or two on each of the adult medical specialties. Most medical students spend only two months of their four years in medical school specifically studying pediatrics.

Internship: The first year of postgraduate training for a new MD. These youngest doctors are called "interns." They've got the MD degree but no license and minimal practical experience. Try to avoid getting sick at a teaching hospital in July, when the new interns start. Also, keep in mind that an "intern" is a first year doctor-in-training; an "internist" is the short name for a doctor of internal medicine (the general physicians who take care of adults.) Though some interns grow up to be internists, don't call your internist an intern.

Residency: This includes the second and third year of postgraduate training after the intern year. Some programs lump the interns and residents together. Often name tags will have a designation including the abbreviation "PGY" for postgraduate year or "PL" for postlaureate year (these mean the same thing.) The number after the PGY or PL is how many years after training. A PGY-1 is an intern; a PL-3 is an experienced third year resident, often called a "senior resident"; a PGY-6 is someone who is really, really sick of being a resident.

Fellowship: Optional training after completing a residency is called a "fellowship", and the physicians at this level of training are "fellows" whether they're men or women. Fellows obtain subspecialty experience in neurology, thoracic surgery, or something like that.

Attendings: Short for "attending physicians," these are doctors who have completed their training and are acting as instructors in a teaching hospital. They are also the physicians who have final responsibility for the patients. Residents report to attendings.

License: A person with an MD or DO degree can apply for a medical license after one year of postgraduate training. A completed residency is not a requirement to hold a medical license, though doctors cannot refer to themselves as "pediatricians" unless they have successfully completed residency training. With a license you can prescribe medicine, set up your own practice, and bill for your services. To keep a medical license valid, most states require proof of participation in continuing medical education courses.

Board certified/eligible: Aspiring pediatricians are considered "board eligible" after successfully completing a pediatric residency program, and may then take the pediatric board examination. Once this exam is passed, the physician is said to be "board certified" and can begin to use the "FAAP" designation. For pediatricians who are now completing training, further board exams and other proof of competency are required every seven years to continue board certification.

FINDING A DREAM PEDIATRICIAN FOR YOUR CHILDREN

Dream doctors are kind. They're skilled listeners, and can pick up the cues of what's said between the lines to know what's really worrying a parent. Children feel at ease around a good pediatrician, so exams are more thorough and enjoyable. If you've found your dream pediatrician, your children will look forward to their visits. You'll be relying on the pediatrician's office, too:

How well is it run? How good is the staff? If their office is poorly run, even great pediatricians won't be able to keep parents happy.

Unfortunately, the skills that make an excellent pediatrician are not necessarily the skills that are cultivated in medical school. Our education is mostly about diseases, germs, and technologic cures. Somewhere in there we're supposed to learn empathy, and somehow keep our sense of humor so we can deal with pediatric patients. Most medical schools and residency training programs pay very little attention to issues of staff management or business, though these areas can be among the most important ways potential patients grow to love or hate their pediatrician's office.

Parents would love to know how to find that perfect pediatrician and perfect office. Though there's no single answer that works 100 percent of the time, there are some insider tips that can get you pointed in the right direction.

Which Office?

Start with the list provided by your insurance company. Most families who have health care insurance through an employer have either a Health Maintenance Organization (HMO) or Preferred Provider Organization (PPO) style plan with a list of "participating providers." If you go outside of this list, you'll end up spending much more money. Even if you've heard of a superb doctor, it's probably not worth the added expense to see a physician that is out of network. These provider lists change frequently, so it's best to get the most up-to-date list possible. Check the insurance company's Web site.

Location is crucial. Your pediatrician's office should be nearby, so you can get there quickly if needed. Most pediatricians are happy to stay open a little later for an end-of-the-day urgent visit, but if you live an hour away you'll end up in the emergency room after your pediatrician's staff heads home. For the same reason, try to find an office that's easy and quick to reach without much traffic. You'll also want to use an office with close parking, especially if you have younger children in car seats and strollers. Those can be a real hassle to get into an elevator after hiking across a big parking lot. Though many physicians set up their offices in busy medical practice complexes, it is often easier to use a pediatric practice that is not part of a cluster of medical buildings near the hospital.

Look at the office hours. If both parents work, it can be especially valuable to have early-morning or late-day appointments available. Regular weekend hours are also nice. Not only are the actual hours important, but you'll want to ask when they

> ☞ **Before considering an individual doctor, look at the practice. Do they take your insurance? Are they convenient? If you aren't comfortable with a practice, look for a different doctor.**

"roll the phones." That is, when do the people who can schedule appointments answer the phones, rather than an answering service.

Offices will have an after-hours policy for emergency situations that arise when the office is closed. The physicians may return urgent calls on their own, or they may join with other pediatric groups to share call responsibilities. Some pediatricians rely on nurses to return most of their calls, and only get on the phone for more dire emergencies or unusual situations that are beyond the expertise of the nurse. Find out who you'll be able to reach in case of an emergency.

Should you choose a large or small practice? There are advantages and disadvantages of each:

- In a smaller or solo practice, you can see the physician who knows you best every time. But if that one physician is ill or on vacation, there may not be seamless coverage.
- Large practices that have multiple locations may shuffle their doctors from office to office on different days, making it difficult to find your own favorite.
- Small offices will scramble to cover the patients of a doctor unexpectedly called away to the hospital. In a larger office, it's more likely that the patients can be seen in a timely manner by a partner.
- The individual physicians in smaller groups are more likely to have better communication and a more cohesive practice philosophy.
- Though a well-run large group can work to avoid miscommunication and missed follow-ups, you're more likely to get consistent follow-through on labs and other issues from a small office where fewer people are involved in making sure things get done.
- Larger offices are more able to invest in the best technology, including newer vaccines, vision and hearing screening equipment, and laboratory instruments.
- Larger offices are more likely to employ an electronic medical record, which can reduce medical errors by making charts more readable and reliable.

Though these practical issues may not seem as important as who the actual doctor is, don't overlook them. A well-run office that's convenient and reliable can be an excellent foundation for a lasting relationship with your pediatrician.

Which Pediatrician?

Pediatricians come in all shapes and personalities. Which one to choose often comes down to personal preference and comfort.

Old versus Young

The stereotype is that older doctors have more years of valuable experience, and younger doctors are more up-to-date on the latest research and techniques. There's some truth in this. Whether you end up favoring youth versus experience, you'll want to work with doctors who keep up on their reading and maintain a healthy curiosity about children's health. Any doctor, young or old, who feels they already know all they need to know is someone you should avoid. If your gut feeling is that you'd prefer a doctor with some grey hairs, go with that; if you think your children would prefer a younger physician, go that route. Either way can be fine, as long as you are confident and comfortable with your pediatrician's skills and experience.

I'm sometimes asked if I have children, or if a pediatrician needs to have children to be competent. Although I've certainly learned a tremendous amount from my own three kids, I think pediatricians who keep their minds open and really watch children will be able to learn what they need to know, even if they don't have children of their own.

Man versus Woman

Most general pediatricians coming out of training are now women, so it's going to get more difficult to find a male pediatrician in the future. If you've got your own comfort zone about who seems more competent, go with your gut. Most younger children don't care whether their doctor is a man or woman, but many teenagers do. Though you may have to change doctors in ten years, don't get too concerned about matching the genders of your baby and your pediatrician.

Personality Types

Some doctors are quiet and thoughtful; some are kind of kooky. Some are quite direct, and don't beat around the bush; some are much more "gentle" in the way they communicate. Some doctors become more emotionally attached to their families and might act more "friendly"; others prefer to maintain a profession detachment. These and many other aspects of a pediatrician's personality may fit better or worse with what you're looking for. Meet a variety of doctors until you find one that "clicks" for you.

Availability

An otherwise excellent pediatrician with commitments to teaching, research, or other matters may not be regularly available. This may matter more to you if your children are younger or have special health needs that require more frequent visits to a doctor who knows them well.

Super Star versus Others in the Practice

Many practices seem to have one or more "super star" pediatricians. These might be the owners, or might be the senior members, or might be the ones with the most likeable personalities. Though you may have heard how superb that individual doctor is, keep in mind that the practice's "super star" is probably the busiest doctor in the group. You'll have extra long waits, and may not be able to get quick appointments easily. One of the lesser known physicians in a group may fit your style just as well, and might work out better in the long run as your main go-to doctor.

How Doctors Dress

The traditional white coat isn't seen much on pediatricians. Though studies have shown that children are *not* more likely to be scared of doctors in white coats, most of us still don't like to wear them. I personally don't wear a tie anymore, either. One good, simple study showed that doctor's neckties can carry disease-causing bacteria. Seen more often in emergency rooms or among specialists who perform surgical procedures, scrubs are popular because they are comfortable, they look cool, they're easy to choose in the morning, and they're free. (Actually, the ones with hospital insignia are not supposed to be free; they're supposed to be worn only in the operating rooms of the hospital. Doctors routinely ignore this. The scrubs with wacky designs that nurses and techs wear are purchased.)

Whatever pediatricians wear, they ought to appear professional and clean. Pediatricians' attire isn't the most important thing, but it will be one way that you'll make your own impression about their competence and professionalism.

If your child has special or chronic health problems, you may want to look for a doctor with particular interest or expertise in that area. Local parent support groups can be a good informal resource for these sorts of referrals, as can physical therapists, specialists, or other people who work with kids who have similar problems. Though you might continue to work with a geneticist as a resource for your child with Down Syndrome, for instance, it would be nice to know that your pediatrician is also familiar and comfortable with working with these kids' special issues.

Do these quotes sound familiar to you? You might have met a doctor like one of these! Every doctor can have bits of every one of these personalities:

- *Dr. Defer:* "Well, what did the other doctor say? You should do that."
- *Dr. Detective:* "I see your baby's diaper has his name written on it, and he's also got his name written on a piece of tape on his back. That means he goes to day care and there was a substitute today."
- *Dr. Entertainer:* "Look at those monkeys in your ear! They're having a picnic!"

- *Dr. Exact:* "At this age, begin feeding your child 12 cheerios between 10 and 11:30 am, followed by an ounce and a half of organic apple juice. You have to introduce solids alphabetically and only on cloudy days."
- *Dr. Experience:* "I've always done it this way, and it always works."
- *Dr. Incisive:* "Do this, now. There's no other way."
- *Dr. Reassuring:* "Don't worry about it! Everyone has one of those."
- *Dr. Refer:* "I'm sending you to the neurologist, orthopedist, and allergist."
- *Dr. Thorough:* (Says very little because the intense and exacting physical exam lasts twenty minutes.)

VETTING US OUT

You've got some good names and you've got some good practices in mind. How do you get the inside story to weed out the potential bad apples?

Friends and neighbors are the best resource for finding out about local doctors. If you have friends with children, ask them about their experiences with nearby pediatric groups. See how enthusiastic they are about their own doctor, or if they have misgivings. You can also get a more honest assessment of waiting times or difficulty in getting appointments from a patient's family than from a doctor's office.

If you can, take advantage of the knowledge of other health care people in your community. Pharmacists take orders from doctors' offices every day, and they know who's organized and on top of things versus who just prescribes the same antibiotic or cold medicine to every single patient. Emergency room nurses know which community doctors take good care of their patients, versus the doctors who are too lazy to return their phone calls. You might get helpful insight from a dentist, orthodontist, physical therapist, optometrist, or another medical specialist. It never hurts to ask, "Who would you choose if you needed a pediatrician for your kids?"

Malpractice claims histories are a matter of public record, and in many states other sorts of disciplinary actions are also reported. You can investigate any physician through www.docboard.org, a nonprofit site that links to individual state medical boards and their claims records. Other Web sites sell combined claims records for a

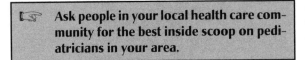

Ask people in your local health care community for the best inside scoop on pediatricians in your area.

fee, which may be useful if you do not know in which states a potential doctor has practiced. Keep in mind that a pediatrician has about a one in three lifetime risk of being targeted in a malpractice lawsuit. Yet doctors who are successfully sued or settle a claim out of court may be excellent physicians guilty of nothing more than bad luck. You may also find that doctors that practice in high-risk specialties or who attract difficult or sick patients will end up with more than their share of lawsuits. Still, if a doctor you are thinking of using has a string of many lawsuits or settlements, you should probably think again.

RED FLAGS? LOOK OUT!

Maybe you're starting to wonder if you've made the wrong choice. There are some signs that mean "steer clear":

- An office that's too busy to help you isn't a place you want to be. If the staff can't take the time to answer your questions or fill out your forms in a reasonable amount of time, then they're too busy to pay attention to the details that are required to practice good medicine. Move on.
- Offices that try to sell you things are taking unfair advantage of their patients. Though some specialties (especially dermatology) may sell specific, hard-to-find items, general pediatric offices should not be health care bazaars. There is always a conflict of interest if someone can make more money by suggesting a certain product; you want to be sure that your pediatrician's judgment is solely based on the health of your children. Be especially wary of the sale of high-priced vitamins or other supplements, which are often part of shady multilevel marketing schemes.
- An unhappy staff or an unhappy doctor means trouble. Sure, anyone can have a bad day once in a while, but if your pediatricians or their staff are not happy at their jobs then you won't be happy as their patients.
- Beware of sloppy records. Doctor's offices should keep good tabs on your medical information, either using neat and organized paper charts or a computer-based record. If you see stacks of charts all over the place with papers falling out, you can bet that they'll have a hard time getting your child's health information organized when it is needed.

For those of you with HMO-style insurance, there is a sneaky trick that some offices may try to use. Using a so-called "capitated" payment schedule, many HMOs pay their participating physicians whether or not patients are actually seen—in other words, they pay the same amount from month to month, whether your child is seen zero, one, or ten times. Doctors who receive capitated payments can make just as much money by seeing these patients less frequently. Be aware that some practices may try to limit their encounters with HMO patients to increase the slots available to those that pay each time they're seen. That can unfairly increase your wait to get an appointment.

Rationing Slots for HMO Patients Can Limit Your Access to the Doctor

Every pediatrician has a certain number of appointment slots each day. For the sake of this example, let's say 50 percent of a practice's patients are enrolled in a capitated HMO called "Choice Health." The practice management may logically declare that 50 percent of the slots should go to Choice Health patients, so that they don't crowd out patients who bring income with every visit. That seems fair enough. But what if those 50 percent HMO patients bring in only 40 percent of the practice's revenue? Should they be limited to only 40 percent of the slots? What if the practice management team decides to become a little more greedy, and limit them to 30 percent of the slots? Remember, because of the HMO payment scheme it is in the interest of the physician's office to decrease the number of encounters with HMO patients. This may not be in the best interests of the patients themselves. If you belong to an HMO and there seems to be a long delay in getting appointments with a certain office, you may have found a place that is more aggressively "rationing" out the HMO slots.

WORKING WITH PARTNERS

Most families choose a small or large group rather than a solo pediatric practitioner, so even if you have a single favorite doctor you may end up having to rely on a partner for an emergency or on a weekend. Try to develop a relationship with a few "back-ups" so your child will feel comfortable even when their favorite doctor is unavailable. Avoid dealing with temporary or "fill-in" doctors, who won't be able to follow through with your issues and might not know your local medical community well. These temps are sometimes called "locum tenets" or just "locums."

Why Do I Get Different Medical Advice When I Speak with Different Doctors?

- Despite our trying to follow the best evidence-based medicine, our judgment is always affected by our own personal experience. If I've had a child have a life-threatening allergic reaction to a certain antibiotic, I'm going to be reluctant to use it on anyone in the future. There's a balance in decision making between the best available evidence and our own experiences with patients regarding what has worked and hasn't worked, or what has been safe and what has led to dangerous side effects.
- A difference in style can lead to differences in practice. One doctor might be very conservative and reluctant to prescribe medicine unless absolutely necessary; another doctor might feel that a prescription is a good way to help parents feel that they're "doing something."
- Sincere differences in medical opinions can be based on a careful consideration of what's known and unknown in medicine. In other words, we certainly don't know everything; two well-read doctors can honestly come to different conclusions.

It can be advantageous to hear two or more differing opinions, especially when the consensus in the medical community is murky.

Look at these as opportunities to learn more by saying "Dr. Smith told me something different. Why are there two opinions on this?" This can help you make a better decision. Good doctors can—and should—occasionally disagree.

FAMILY OR FRIENDS AS DOCTORS

You might have neighbors or family members who are pediatricians. Some of us don't feel comfortable routinely treating children that we know personally—it can be difficult to make objective decisions. Ask any potential pediatricians that you know personally how they feel about seeing your family as patients.

Even if they're not your doctor, you might be able to get some "friendly advice" on the side from a family or friend medical resource. For minor issues this can be a big help, but let your pediatrician's office know if any medications were prescribed. If there's something significant going on, it is better to get a thorough evaluation at a routine visit than to rely on offhand or informal advice from a well-meaning friend.

WHAT TO DO IF YOU'RE NOT HAPPY

Remember: you aren't married to your pediatrician, and you don't have to ask for a divorce. You may have had a bad medical experience, or you just might feel that your personalities don't fit well together. Perhaps your child has just decided that one particular doctor is fearsome. If you're not happy, for whatever reason, it is perfectly fine for you to move on. You can try another pediatrician in the practice, or move to another practice entirely. If changing practices, have a copy of the records sent over, or bring them yourself. The most critical part of the record will usually be the immunization history; get a copy of that for yourself to keep whenever you change offices.

If you have only minor quibbles, feel free to point out your concerns to your pediatrician. Sometimes this sort of feedback can lead to an improvement. But your job is not to fix a pediatric practice. You should be happy and comfortable with your child's pediatrician.

A pediatrician is the best individual to help most families make health decisions for their children. But many other individuals are highly trained, essential resources. In the next chapter, we'll look past the pediatrician to find out about the best players for the rest of the health care team.

2

THE REST OF YOUR CHILD'S HEALTH CARE TEAM

To give the best care, your child's physician will need help: skilled and patient nurses, physician extenders, and specialists. Though most children rely on a pediatrician as their main physician, some families work with a qualified family practitioner or general practitioner instead. Knowing the inside story on the people who work with your pediatrician will help you choose the best team to help take care of your child.

OTHER DOCTORS

Like pediatricians, family physicians have a three year residency to learn the practical aspects of patient care after medical school. Though pediatricians only concentrate on children, family physicians also study adult medicine, obstetrics, gynecology, and minor surgery. They do not typically spend much training time on inpatient or intensive care unit medicine. Although there is certainly appeal in being able to take your entire family to the same doctor, our concentration on children's issues gives pediatricians more training and experience in dealing with childhood health problems, especially issues that are rare.

Physicians who call themselves "general practitioners" (GPs) are becoming less common. They've probably completed only one year of residency after medical school, and do not have any board exams or other professional qualifiers to ensure that they stay competent beyond minimal state licensing standards. Though in past generations the neighborhood GP had been a valuable source of solid health expertise, the sheer volume of new information about diseases and therapeutics has run ahead of many GP's relatively brief training.

PHYSICIAN EXTENDERS AND NURSES

The phrase "physician extender" refers to nonphysicians who nonetheless have strong qualifications and training to diagnose and treat many common conditions of childhood. Most extenders are either Physician Assistants (PAs) or Nurse Practitioners (NPs) who have completed master's degree coursework and clinical internships. In most states they can prescribe medications, perform medical procedures, and in other ways perform duties traditionally done by doctors. Though they must be supervised by a physician, in many circumstances they perform independently. Well-trained extenders can handle many common and not-so-common problems that fall into their expertise and background. Your pediatrician's office may employ one or more extenders to do both sick and well visits, or to see patients in the hospital. Traditionally, extenders are thought to be able to spend more time with patients, which can certainly be a plus for many families looking for comprehensive care.

Throughout this book, I'll refer to the person taking care of your children as their pediatrician. What I really mean is "pediatrician, extender, family practitioner, or whoever else is acting in the role of your child's doctor." I don't mean to exclude these other qualified people; I just find all of that typing awkward.

You'll usually call the people in the office who bring back your child, do measurements, and give immunizations "nurse." But you should know that there are different levels of training for what are commonly called nurses, and that some of the people working in that role aren't really nurses at all. The best trained nurses usually seen in doctors' offices are Registered Nurses, or "RNs". They've completed a two to four year course of academic and clinical training, and have passed a national licensing exam. One step below in training is the Licensed Practical Nurse, or "LPN." They've usually had up to eighteen months of training, usually at a vocational school or community college, and must also pass their own licensing examination. The least trained of all go by several names, including "nurse technicians," "nurse aids," "techs," or "medical assistants." Their training may last only a few months, and genuine nurses might chafe at their being lumped in with the nurses in a medical office. They are not licensed and are not required to pass any exams, though some states do require medical assistants to pass certification exams if they want to perform certain procedures. Many pediatric practices rely on these non-nurses to do traditional nursing duties because they can be hired for less pay. Whichever your pediatrician chooses to hire, you should expect anyone working in the office to be well-trained and friendly, with a confident ability to handle most situations. More importantly, nurses or medical assistants need to know when they are in over their head so they can quickly ask for help.

Some pediatrician's offices have nurses in specific roles:

- The Head Nurse is usually the senior, most trusted nurse. She takes care of nurse staffing issues.
- A triage nurse decides how quickly a patient needs to be seen by the doctor, whether they're in person or over the phone.
- Phone nurses are devoted to returning calls, and usually take care of forms and other administrative tasks.

Keep your eye out to discover if your pediatrician has one "personal nurse," that is, a single nurse that he or she works with every day. If your pediatrician does have a single nurse who acts as a professional assistant, that's the best person to try to reach on the phone if you need questions answered or a favor from your doctor.

THE STAFF

While working with your pediatrician you'll also rely on receptionists, insurance clerks, and other "back-office" assistants. They'll help you make appointments, take care of referrals, and make sure bills get paid. Larger medical offices will often have an office manager or business manager in charge of staff and office procedures. A happy and efficient staff can make working with your doctor a pleasure; an incompetent or grouchy staff should send you running away from even the best pediatrician's office.

> ☞ **You're choosing more than a doctor when you choose your pediatrician. Look for a happy and competent staff, too.**

If you do have a problem with a nurse or any staff member, be sure to bring it up with your doctor. We want to stay in business, and we need to hear the good and the bad so we can keep a good staff in place.

THE SPECIALISTS

Although they're not used as commonly as in adult medicine, pediatricians occasionally refer to specialists to confirm a diagnosis or to help with the ongoing management of a chronic problem. Specialists are also able to do diagnostic and therapeutic procedures, like allergy skin testing or a hernia repair, which are beyond the expertise of pediatricians. In this section, I'll reveal the insider tips on the different kinds of specialists, reviewing how to choose one, and what problems each is best at managing.

How to Choose a Specialist

If you are in a managed care plan, it is usually best to start with the list of in-network physicians. Although you may have heard of a super-genius specialist, if that name isn't on your list you can probably find someone just as good that is in the network. Use your pediatrician as your specialist resource, even if a referral is not required. Your pediatrician knows most of the specialists in your area, and can steer you to the best ones with the expertise to address your concerns. If your child has an especially urgent problem, your pediatrician's office may be able to get you a quicker appointment, but keep in mind that what may seem like a dire emergency to you may be fairly routine to a specialist. They will usually squeeze in an "emergency" appointment only if delay will physically harm your child, not just because of parental anxiety.

Community versus University Specialists

Some specialists practice through a university, often at the university hospital. Traditionally, these specialists are thought to be more familiar with the latest research and more devoted to the hottest technology. They have access to the research facilities of the university, and mingle professionally with other academics. But from a practical point of view, dealing with university specialists is a hassle. It is usually more difficult to park, more difficult to get through on the phone, and more difficult to get an appointment than with community specialists. Increasingly, though, the distinction is blurring between the university and community specialists. Often the university has offsite clinics that are run more like private practices and less like frustrating bureaucratic institutions. Community specialists have always trained alongside their academic counterparts, and can remain actively involved with the local university medical community. Work with your pediatrician to decide if a trip to a university medical center is needed.

Genuine Pediatric versus Adult Specialists

In many specialties there are few practitioners who are solely devoted to children. This is especially true in smaller communities. Usually, the adult specialists can handle children, but some situations call for a true pediatric specialist:

- A very young child
- A complex or rare problem
- A problem that requires technical expertise specific for children

Given a choice, I would usually opt for a pediatric specialist if one is available. Again, work with your pediatrician to decide what kind of specialist is best for your child's specific problem.

Allergists and Immunologists

Allergists diagnose and treat allergic conditions such as hay fever, asthma, food allergies, and eczema. Many of them also become involved with the diagnosis and treatment of immune deficiency states [except AIDS (Acquired Immune Deficiency Syndrome), which belongs to the infectious disease specialists]. As allergies are so common, your pediatrician should be adept at diagnosing and treating most of them. But if your child is not responding to the medicines your pediatrician is comfortable using, or if you want your child tested to identify specific allergic triggers, an allergist is for you.

> ☞ **Even if your insurance doesn't require a formal referral, rely on your pediatrician as the best resource to suggest the specialist that you need.**

Most allergists see adults and kids, and that is fine. If your child has a specific, severe immune deficiency (these are rare), you should probably be working with a university-affiliated pediatric immune specialist.

Allergists approach allergic disease by first identifying specific triggers. A careful history, sometimes backed up by focused testing, will usually reveal what environmental factors are triggering the allergy. Avoidance of those triggers is essential. Allergists also use a variety of medicines that general pediatricians also prescribe, including antihistamines and topical steroids. Furthermore, allergists are trained to administer immunotherapy, or "allergy shots." These can involve years of frequent injections, but when other methods fail allergy shots can alleviate the symptoms of difficult allergy patients.

There is a mystifying list of other issues for which some people seek an allergist's assistance. These include school problems, behavioral problems, chronic pain, or other vague complaints that are not allergy-based. An ethical allergist will not claim to be able to help with these things, and should gently steer those without illness caused by allergy toward other resources. Note that allergy itself can cause difficulty in school, if for instance chronic congestion leads to sleepless nights and poor school focus; but without evidence of clear allergic symptoms there is no role for allergy testing or allergy treatment in individuals with these sorts of complaints.

Cardiologists

Work with a cardiologist who specializes in children if your pediatrician identifies signs of possible heart disease, including frequent or severe fainting, an unusual heart murmur, or palpitations. In pediatrics, important heart disease is usually present at birth, caused by a problem with the development of the heart. These heart defects are often diagnosed well before the babies are born by routine prenatal ultrasounds.

Most children who have an occasional, ordinary faint do not need a cardiologist; likewise, common murmurs that are heard in many children are completely normal. Your pediatrician should feel comfortable and confident in screening these problems to avoid the extra anxiety and expense of specialty referral.

A common referral to pediatric cardiology is a child with chest pain, but children with chest pain almost never have anything wrong with their heart. A cardiology evaluation would be warranted if chest pain is always triggered by exercise or is accompanied by certain red flags: palpitations, shortness of breath, or fainting.

Dentists

Physicians get remarkably little training in oral health, so we have a low threshold for referring tooth, mouth, or other oral problems to the dentist or oral surgeon. By age three or so, every child should have a dental exam. Some community dentists do a fine job seeing both adults and kids, while other dentists prefer to only see adults. There are pediatric dentists who can do a superb job with even the most frightened children, but most kids will do fine with a family dentist.

Dermatologists

There are few genuine "pediatric dermatologists," and many general dermatologists do a good job with children. But most skin conditions should almost always first be seen by a pediatrician. We see a lot of rashes, and can easily identify and treat conditions like acne, eczema, diaper rash, poison ivy, and rashes caused by viruses. Dermatologists are most useful for kids who have difficult-to-treat chronic rashes, including severe forms of eczema or acne, or children whose workup might require a biopsy.

One very common reason for a dermatology referral is warts, or a similar rash called "molluscum." These can be difficult and frustrating to treat, and though they are only cosmetic they can lead to a lot of anxiety. Try your pediatrician's favorite inexpensive and painless methods to eradicate them first. Dermatologists more often rely on techniques that might be more painful and costly, and may not be any more effective.

Emergency Room Physicians

It's never a single room anymore, and most hospitals now call it the "Emergency Department." But the doctors who work there are still known as ER physicians. They are cool characters, ready to handle a crisis. Because they don't rely on repeat business and don't usually develop lasting relationships with their patients, ER doctors may not be the warmest and fuzziest of pediatricians. Keep in mind that they're there to take care of the sickest kids first, which may have nothing to do with the order in which families arrived.

Though you won't really have the ability to choose which ER physician sees your child, ask your pediatrician which hospital has the best-staffed ER so you know where to go if a serious health issue comes up while your pediatrician's office is closed.

Endocrinologists

The initial workup for most suspected endocrinology problems, including thyroid disease and diabetes, should be started by the pediatrician; referral to an endocrinologist is needed if the tests show one of these conditions, and is unnecessary if the tests are negative. A child with poor growth or delayed puberty can likewise have an initial hormone evaluation done be a pediatrician, with quick referral if the tests show a likely endocrine problem. Referral is usually indicated even if the tests are normal in a child who is truly very different from his or her peers in these areas.

A growing source of referrals to endocrinologists is the vast number of overweight children. Despite extensive testing that is sometimes insisted on by parents very few of these children have an identifiable hormone imbalance causing their weight problems. A general pediatrician should be able to screen the most severe kids with weight problems for endocrine issues that require specialty referral, including those that are at risk for diabetes.

ENT (Ear, Nose, and Throat) Specialist

True "pediatric ENTs" are hard to find, and many general adult ENTs do fine with kids. If you need an ENT referral, ask your pediatrician for a specific name or two, as different problems require a different level of expertise and training. By far the most common diagnosis prompting ENT referral is a child with frequent or difficult-to-treat ear infections. In the United States, the second most-often performed surgical procedure is the placement of plastic tubes to drain persistently or recurrently infected ears. (For the curious, the most-often performed surgical procedure in children is routine neonatal circumcision.)

In the past, ENTs were often called to perform tonsillectomies for children with frequent sore throats or "big" tonsils. We now know that most of these procedures are unnecessary and potentially harmful. Surgical removal of tonsils should be considered for frequent throat infections *only* if they're proven to be caused by strep bacteria; the procedure is unlikely to be of any benefit to children who are having frequent viral infections. Tonsillectomy should also be considered for the treatment of children whose large tonsils prevent them from breathing while they sleep, a condition called "Obstructive Sleep Apnea." Without these indications, tonsillectomy should be a very rare procedure; your pediatrician should know to avoid referral to ENTs that are too quick to recommend surgery.

If you are referred to an ENT for frequent ear infections or strep throats, bring a "problem list" from your pediatrician. Though the ENT will not need the details in your entire pediatric chart, she will want to review how many infections have occurred, the dates, and how they were treated. This should be available on a short form created from your pediatric records.

ENTs can also help with problematic or frequent sinus infections, nosebleeds, vocal cord or upper airway problems, and hearing loss.

Gastroenterologists (GI)

I rarely refer patients to GI physicians, though GI complaints are so common. Many children have abdominal pain, and very few of these require the input of a specialist to help. A general pediatrician should also be adept at handling chronic constipation, diarrhea, and poor weight gain. Very few of these children have anything complex. In fact, the pediatrician's approach, which should stress the whole family situation rather than high-tech tests and procedures, is more suited to help the vast majority of patients with GI complaints.

That being said, a GI physician's input can be very valuable for children with symptoms like severe, chronic abdominal pain, recurrent vomiting, or persistent diarrhea, especially if these symptoms are accompanied by weight loss. Also, a pediatrician's screening blood and stool tests might show abnormalities that warrant a specialist referral. A gastroenterologist can also perform an endoscopy and obtain biopsies to confirm a suspected diagnosis. Any child with a serious, chronic gut condition such as Crohn Disease or cystic fibrosis should have ongoing followup by a dedicated pediatric gastroenterologist.

General Surgeons

Here, I'm talking about general surgeons who specialize in children. They may become involved in your child's care in an emergency, after an accident, or during an ER presentation for a possible appendicitis. You may also be referred electively for evaluation of a hernia, or a cyst that has to be removed. I encourage families to seek the help of surgeon trained with children if this is possible, even in an emergency situation. Pediatric surgeons have at least two extra years of training specifically working with pediatric patients, and are better at using smaller instruments and smaller incisions. They are also probably better at communicating with parents, which is a crucial issue during the care of a potentially very sick child.

Gynecologists

Adolescents can work with any gynecologist—though I recommend moms respect their daughter's preferences. An adolescent may prefer to see only a female gynecologist, and may have very strong feelings about seeing the same gynecologist as her mother. Your daughter should be comfortable feeling that she has her "own" woman's doctor. Although a chaperone (usually a nurse, and always a woman) will be present during any examination, ask your daughter in advance whether she prefers mom to stay in the room. Very few fathers would even think of sharing this experience!

It is uncommon for young girls to require an evaluation by a gynecologist, but if your child needs this sort of exam ask your pediatrician for a referral to a gynecologist with specific training and experience with children. Although a one year fellowship in pediatric gynecology is available, most practicing pediatric gynecologists have done their extra training through less formal venues. It takes special experience, equipment, and temperament to perform a gynecologic exam on a young girl, and most communities have just one or two gynecologists who can do this. To avoid pain and trauma, sometimes the exam requires brief general anesthesia.

Hospitalists

This is a relatively new specialty, but one that will certainly be growing. Hospitalists are pediatricians who only take care of hospitalized patients. They may have additional specialty training in any other field (pulmonary, neurology, or anything else), or they may have only general pediatric training. Many pediatric practices in urban and suburban settings have decided that if one of their patients is hospitalized, their own doctors will not follow them in the hospital. Rather, they'll be taken care of by the full time hospitalist service. At discharge, the hospitalist should contact the usual pediatrician to hand back care by reviewing the case and any plans that were made.

Advantages of using a hospitalist:

- They're in the hospital for more hours—in some cases twenty-four hours a day. Evaluations and decisions can be made at any time, rather than just once or twice a day when the traditional pediatrician's rounds take place.
- Hospitalists spend all of their time working with hospital-level problems, and may remain more up to date on these sorts of issues than the community pediatrician who infrequently is in charge of hospitalized kids.
- Hospital care has become more and more complex. The kids are sicker than ever because the threshold for hospitalization has risen. These days, you've got to be very ill to end up in the hospital! At the same time, the average length of stay has fallen, so that decisions have to be made more quickly. More and more high technology tests are available, and these need to be understood and used correctly. Many hospitals have installed computer based medical records that are difficult to learn if they are not used every day. Some community-based general pediatricians may be becoming less technically able to care for hospitalized patients on their own.

Disadvantages of using a hospitalist:

- The hospitalist will not know your child and your family. In my experience, kids who are ill are very happy to see a familiar doctor. Even burly and surly teenagers have thanked me for coming in to see them when they're sick. Familiarity, comfort, and confidence in a well-known doctor are powerful feelings, especially when a child is fearful and ill.
- Follow-up can be fragmented, especially if specialists become involved. With a complex or serious illness, it really is best if a single physician stays involved and keeps track of everything that's going on, whether the patient is in or out of the hospital.

Whether your hospitalized child ends up on your pediatrician's service or on the hospitalists' will depend on the policy of your pediatrician's office. Unfortunately, many pediatric offices are forced to make a decision on this issue in financial terms. Because we see so few inpatients, it does not make economic sense for us to spend time in the hospital. In other words, we'll collect more revenue by spending the time that would have been involved with inpatient care seeing more patients in our offices.

If you have strong feelings about whether you want your own pediatricians to take care of hospitalized children, ask about their office policy in advance. Should your child end up on a hospitalist's service, ensure the best follow-up by asking the inpatient doctor to call your own physician personally on the phone. Bring copies of all hospital records, including laboratory reports, tests, and x-rays, to your own pediatrician for follow-up care. Keep records of any specialists that come to see you, and be sure to ask each one if you need to follow-up with them or your general pediatrician after discharge. Hospitalists practice good medicine, but when you work with them you'll need to be more thorough about making sure your own pediatrician gets the whole story.

Infectious Disease Specialists

Pediatricians see a tremendous amount of infectious disease, and rarely need a specialist's help to diagnose or treat these sorts of problems. But a pediatric infectious disease specialist can be a great resource for the treatment of chronic infections (especially HIV or chronic hepatitis), rare and serious infections (like meningitis), or in the evaluation of a child with a prolonged unexplained fever. Pediatric infectious disease specialists can also be helpful in the prevention, recognition, and management of diseases encountered during foreign travel.

Neurologists

The most common reason for neurology referral is headaches, though certainly most headaches can be diagnosed and managed by a good pediatrician. A neurologist can be helpful if first line therapy and trigger avoidance fails, especially for severe migraine headaches. Neurologists are also very good resources for children with recurrent seizures, though a pediatrician should do fine taking care of the evaluation following a single seizure, especially if the evaluation confirms that the seizure is unlikely to recur. Neurologists can also be helpful in the evaluation of developmental problems and suspected cerebral palsy, along with a wide variety of rarer conditions.

Neurologists are often consulted for school problems and ADD, though in most cases a general pediatrician or mental health expert would be more appropriate. Sometimes insurance companies "carve out" mental health benefits, refusing to pay for a psychiatrist. A family may feel forced into care for mental illness like bipolar disorder by a neurologist even though a psychiatrist has more appropriate training and experience.

Neurosurgeons

The only common patient referred from a pediatrician to a neurosurgeon is an infant with a flattened head. Many infants are born with molding of their skull into a cone kind of shape to facilitate childbirth. The head should regain a nice round shape within a few weeks. In some children, especially those that are temperamentally less active, heads can tend to flatten again. Heads are never perfectly round, but your pediatrician should watch the shape and size of your child's head at well child visits. If there is more than mild skull flattening that does not improve with some simple home maneuvers the pediatrician can teach you, than a neurosurgical consultation may be appropriate. Very, very few of these children need surgery, but the neurosurgeons can help with nonsurgical treatment of this problem using a custom-made helmet device.

Ophthalmologists

My bias is to refer, immediately, any child with a suspected eye or vision problem to a pediatric ophthalmologist. It is especially important to quickly refer any child with crossed eyes, suspected lazy eye, or an unusual color to the pupil to a pediatric ophthalmologist. Vision is very important, and though a community pediatrician should carefully and thoroughly screen for potential eye problems at every well visit is it difficult to do a comprehensive eye exam on a child. Any hint of a potentially serious eye problem warrants referral.

Everyday eye problems that can be easily addressed by your pediatrician include the initial evaluation and management of a pink eye, minor eye scratches or injuries, and intermittent crossing of the eyes in a baby less than six months of age.

Orthopedists (Orthopedic Surgeons)

Orthopedists treat acute, severe injuries, as well as chronic pain in limbs and joints. Your general pediatrician can often help with these issues as well, though most pediatricians are limited by not having access to their own x-ray equipment, and not having the expertise to definitively treat a serious injury. If your child is a serious athlete, you should work with an orthopedist with a particular interest in sports medicine for sports related injuries and pain. Related specialists, called sports medicine physicians, have similar training in the management of sports injuries, but they lack the surgical training of the orthopedists.

Some insider tips can help decide if your pediatrician, an orthopedist, or an emergency room physician is needed when your child is injured:

- For a sudden, dramatic injury where there is obviously a fracture: try to immobilize the limb, and go straight to the nearest emergency room. This would include any injury where the limb is bent or any bone is sticking out. Don't give the child anything to eat or drink, as sedation may be necessary.
- For a sudden injury followed by pain or swelling: try to immobilize the limb or joint to prevent more motion, and apply ice. If the pain isn't too intense, wait for an hour or so to see how the child does before immediately seeking care. If you already know an orthopedist, or have an orthopedic office nearby, call and see if you can get a quick appointment. Alternatively, go to a local urgent care center where a physician can evaluate your child and perform an x-ray. If a sudden injury occurs and pain or swelling persists, an x-ray is probably needed.
- One special type of injury that is common and well suited to pediatric care is a toddler age child who refuses to move an arm. If this occurs after the child has fallen out of bed it is usually a broken clavicle, which can easily be managed by a general pediatrician after x-rays. If this occurs after anyone jerked the arm of the child, it is probably a "nursemaid's elbow", which your pediatrician should be able to quickly fix without any x-rays. For a young child who won't move an arm, call your pediatrician for advice first.

- For more mild or chronic pain, either without any preceding injury or following a relatively minor injury, most pediatricians can do a good job in assessment and treatment. You should also visit your pediatrician first for limb pain that goes along with other symptoms, like fever or a rash.

Psychiatrists

Psychiatrists are medical doctors trained to diagnose and treat mental illness. They primarily treat patients with medicine, though some also perform psychotherapy (talk therapy). For issues including anxiety, bipolar illness, and obsessive compulsive disorder, the most effective therapy is usually going to include medicine, so involvement of a psychiatrist is more essential.

Some health care plans "carve out" mental health benefits, refusing to pay for services rendered by psychiatrists, psychologists, or mental health counselors. See Chapter 14 for additional information about ways to get the most mental health coverage out of your insurance plan.

Psychologists

Unlike psychiatrists, psychologists cannot prescribe medicine. They can be very helpful with the assessment and treatment of many problems of childhood, including school difficulties, divorce, gender identity problems, social phobias, behavioral challenges, and many other problems. They also often work collaboratively with psychiatrists in the treatment of problems like attention deficit disorder, depression, and anxiety.

Many people are trained to provide counseling for children, including psychologists, licensed counselors, and social workers. Training often involves masters-level degrees, and many practicing psychologists carry the title "Doctor" because they have completed a Ph.D. program. Licensing requirements vary by state authorities, who regulate who can call themselves a "counselor" or "therapist." As psychologists and other therapists often develop specific interests and expertise, it's best to work with your pediatrician to find someone in your area who has the best background to tackle your child's problem.

Pulmonologists

Pulmonary specialists deal with lungs, and their main bread-and-butter issue is recurrent wheezing, or asthma. If your asthmatic child requires more than two medicines to stay symptom free, a pulmonologist's evaluation can be especially helpful. These lung specialists are also are involved in the care of premature babies with chronic lung disease, and can help with the evaluation of a child who seems to tire out easily or gets short of breath during sports.

Radiologists

Like anesthesiologists and pathologists, radiologists work "behind the scenes," and are not typically chosen by the patient. But whether or not you get an accurate diagnosis depends on the quality of the equipment, the technician, and the radiologist who interprets the film.

Donnie had been diagnosed with pneumonia while traveling out of town and mom brought his chest x-ray with him for followup for me to review. He was doing fine—no more cough, no more fever—but his x-ray was a mess! Though I'm not a radiologist, he clearly had several dense blobs next to his spine on both of the two x-rays that I was looking at. I didn't want to alarm mom, so I told her I'd just bounce these off of a local radiologist. The first one I found at the children's hospital glanced at them and said "That's really something. Probably cancer." He suggested I have the child sedated for a few hours to do an MRI scan of his entire brain and spine. I then found a radiologist who I've known for years—an excellent, smart guy who always has time for my questions. He looked at the exact same films and said "I don't believe any of this." He thought the films were poorly done on poor equipment, and said the first thing he would do is just repeat the x-ray. On the repeat films, all of the blobs were gone! And I never did mention the "C" word to mom. What makes this story especially memorable to me is that he didn't in fact have pneumonia on the x-rays, either!

To get the most reliable results from radiology tests, try to work with a pediatric center. Their equipment is better set up for smaller people, and their technicians will be more experienced in using the least radiation needed to get a good film. Follow any instructions carefully regarding preparation, whether your child needs an empty stomach or a bowel preparation regimen. If specialist follow-up is anticipated, bring a copy of the films with you. And don't be afraid to ask your pediatrician to review the film, or bounce it off of their favorite radiologist, if something unexpected comes up.

One other pitfall: if your child is evaluated in an emergency room or urgent care center after hours, there is a good chance that any x-rays will be read by the ER doctor rather than a radiologist. This is OK, as ER docs are seldom going to overlook anything truly important. But find out before you leave if anyone else will be reading and interpreting the film, and make sure that a copy of this report is reviewed by your pediatrician. In most cases, a formal x-ray reading will be done by a radiologist, and their report will need to be reviewed for any important findings that may have been missed.

Renal Specialists (Nephrologists)

Most cities have just a couple of pediatric kidney specialists, as these problems are so rare in children. Most referrals are done on the basis of screening urine tests done at well checks, which may show some blood or protein in the urine. Though the majority of these kids are fine, the appearance of blood or protein in the urine may be an early warning sign of kidney disease. Most pediatricians will begin the evaluation on their own, and refer kids who have other suspicious findings on follow-up tests. Children with high blood pressure may also need an evaluation by a kidney specialist.

Rheumatologists

One of the rarest pediatric specialists, these physicians should be involved in the care of children with rheumatoid arthritis, lupus, scleroderma, and other inflammatory diseases of joints and skin. Unfortunately, many children are referred to rheumatologists for vague chronic pain who are otherwise normal. Kids with body pains who have no swollen or red joints, no fevers, and normal blood tests are very unlikely to have any sort of inflammatory disease. They do not need a rheumatologist's input, though the reassurance of this sort of specialist can be therapeutic itself. For children with chronic pain whose medical evaluation is normal, a better resource for referrals would be a psychologist, psychiatrist, or physical therapist. Families will sometimes fight a psychological referral vehemently, insisting that their child visit every possible "medical" specialist first; thus rheumatologists become involved, who then send the children onward to physical therapy and counseling.

Another common source of referrals to rheumatology are children who have a positive blood test called an "ANA." This test is incorrectly considered a screening test for rheumatologic disease such as lupus. Unfortunately, the ANA is a terrible test to screen for these problems. Positive ANA tests are found in many children who are absolutely normal. If your child has had a positive ANA but does not have other objective evidence of rheumatologic disease such as swollen joints, peculiar rashes, or blood in the urine, you should question why the ANA test was done in the first place. ANA tests done on children who have pain without other problems are much more likely to be misleading than helpful in arriving at a diagnosis.

Urologists

Urologists are surgeons trained to operate on the urinary system, from the kidneys to the bladder to the urethra. They also are involved in surgical issues with male genitalia, such as undescended testicles and circumcision issues. Most kids with bedwetting should be handled by their own general pediatrician, but if other issues are present like daytime wetting or especially anxious parents, a urologist's evaluation can be helpful. Urologists are also relied on to help with the management of persistent or severe vesicoureteral reflux (sometimes called "kidney reflux"), which is a common cause of urinary tract infections in young children and babies.

Plastic Surgeons

Plastic surgeons work on cosmetic issues like birthmarks and reconstructive surgery after accidents, and also on the repair of birth defects like cleft palates.

Your pediatrician may suggest a referral to a plastic surgeon after a severe burn or a wound that is not healing well.

Parents sometimes wonder if their child's minor laceration needs to be repaired by a plastic surgeon rather than a general ER physician or their own pediatrician. Keep in mind that ER physicians have extensive experience with wound repair, and will probably do just as good a job as a plastic surgeon. Also, the plastic surgeon can always reevaluate and fix up an old scar later. Although you can insist that a plastic surgeon do the closure of a wound while you are waiting in the ER, this will usually dramatically increase your wait time and is rarely necessary unless it is suggested by the ER physician.

Other Nondoctor Specialists

Occupational therapists, physical therapists, and speech therapists work with children who have problems with age-appropriate activities like playing, walking, or communicating. Their training is usually on a master's degree level, requiring national board exams as well as state licensing requirements that can include ongoing coursework. Some children have issues that overlap between these therapists, and end up working with two or three of these practitioners simultaneously. Many states have "early intervention" programs to identify young children with developmental problems so they can begin these services when they are younger.

Occupational Therapists

Most children learn the ordinary skills of childhood on their own: playing, taking care of themselves, using their hands to write, and getting along with others. Occupational therapists—called "OTs"—help children who are having trouble with these important activities. Children are often referred to an OT if they have developmental delays, trouble with dressing or grooming, or difficulties with coordination.

OTs can also help children with sensory defensiveness. These kids seem overwhelmed by their own senses of touch, sight, and hearing. They have trouble getting through an ordinary day because of loud noises, bright lights, or tags in their clothing that tickle their skin. A related condition, called "sensory integration dysfunction," is a somewhat controversial area that has become a large part of many pediatric OT practices. Children with sensory integration dysfunction are said to have trouble coordinating their interactions with the outside world. Unfortunately, the diagnostic and therapeutic interventions that are being used for this condition have not been well validated, and have not been shown to be effective for the broad categories of children who often seek referral: children with attention problems, autism, learning disabilities, or developmental problems. If you feel your child would benefit from OT for sensory integration dysfunction, you should pick well-defined goals and targets for therapy. If the therapy is helping achieve these tangible goals in a reasonable amount of time, continue the therapy. OTs can certainly help children with muscle disorders or other problems with the nervous system that cause movement or sensory difficulties, but not every child who is having social or school difficulties requires an OT.

Physical Therapists

There is quite a bit of overlap between occupational and physical therapy in children, but one quick rule of thumb is that OTs tend to look at the functioning of the upper body (especially the hands), while physical therapists (PTs) are more concerned with the trunk and lower body. PTs are excellent resources for children who because of illness, trauma, or developmental problems have trouble with rolling, sitting, walking, or running. They can help children with weak muscles or trouble balancing, or children who need assistance with range-of-motion issues related to sports injuries or other trauma. Physical therapy is also an essential part of the treatment of any child with chronic pain or fatigue.

Speech Therapists

Any problem with the functioning of the mouth falls into the realm of a speech therapist (ST): speaking, eating, or drinking. STs can help babies who are having trouble making the transition to solid foods, or older children who have a significant or worsening stutter. School age children with poor articulation or who substitute the wrong letter sounds (W for R, for example) are good candidates for speech therapy, as are child whose speech development has been affected by hearing problems.

Pharmacists

Your pharmacist is an overlooked source of good health advice. Pharmacists have extensive training in the use of medications and may well know more about drug interactions and side effects than your doctor. In addition, pharmacists know a lot of very practical information about how to use medicines while saving money: which pills can be split, and which medications come in generic forms. Once pharmacists get to know your family, they'll be especially good at spotting errors or misunderstandings—they'll know, for instance, which of your children needs asthma medicine versus which is allergic to penicillin. And the advice and expertise of the pharmacist is free!

There are two kinds of pharmacies: local, family-owned places versus the chains. Which one you use is a matter of personal preference, though there are some unique advantages of each:

- Smaller local pharmacies often have a larger variety of items, and are very willing to quickly order in whatever item you want. The big chains tend to carry the entire lines of the big manufacturers' products, but leave out the smaller makers of more "niche" products.
- Larger chains are usually less expensive for staple items, and are more likely to have sales and discount cards.

- If you fill your prescription though a chain, you can usually get refills at any other location. Dealing with a small local pharmacy won't give you that flexibility. Smaller outlets are also less likely to have extensive weekend or twenty-four-hour service.
- Smaller pharmacies will be more willing to "compound" items—in pediatrics, this means they can make a liquid out of a medicine that only comes in pills.
- Large chain outlets are more likely to accept a wide variety of prescription insurance plans—but don't assume that the mom-and-pop pharmacy won't take your insurance.
- At a small family owned pharmacy, you're more likely to always see the same pharmacist. This is the best way to make a beneficial long term relationship.

To Choose Your Health Care Team: Ask for Your Pediatrician's Help

Pediatricians are your best source for information on which local specialists have the expertise your child needs. We know which specialists are friendly and accommodating, versus the ones who never return phone calls. Even if your insurance doesn't require a referral, you should work with your pediatrician to choose the best specialist for your child.

In these first two chapters we've looked at the people who've dedicated their careers to the health of your children. You'll be happiest with your own pediatric practice if you look not only for the best doctor but also for the best nurses and staff. Are they patient and friendly, and most importantly are they glad to see you and your children? You can recognize people who are genuinely good at working with kids if they can make your children smile even when they're sick. That's the best way to know if you've found a good home for pediatric care.

3

WHAT EVERY PEDIATRICIAN SHOULD KNOW

You've chosen your pediatrician. She's kind and friendly, she's good with kids, and she has a well run and convenient office. But how can you be sure she really knows what she's doing? Has she kept up on the latest research and findings, and does she try to follow the best evidence-based guidelines for your child's care?

Though there is no single test of clinical competence, there are a few ways to confirm that your pediatrician is on the ball. Pediatricians should be board certified, or at least "board eligible" if they've only recently completed their training. Board certified doctors have passed their national licensing boards, and have continued to demonstrate their competence through ongoing continuing medical education classes and periodic recertification boards. "Board eligible" means that a residency has been completed, but the board exam either hasn't been taken yet, or hasn't been passed yet. A pediatrician who has been in practice for more than a year but has not yet passed the board exam has some explaining to do. Although there may be a more innocent story, chances are that the newly minted pediatrician failed the board exam.

Another way to ensure that your pediatrician has kept up with new medical information is to confirm that they are familiar with the recommendations from their own mainstream professional organization. The American Academy of Pediatrics (AAP) is the largest professional organization for pediatricians, and almost all board certified pediatricians in the Unites States belong to this group. Most of us use the professional designation "FAAP" after our "MD" or "DO" degrees, indicating that we are "fellows" of the academy. The AAP develops policy statements on health issues based on the best available evidence. They are written by committees of experts, reviewed by peers, re-reviewed by an executive committee, and re-re-reviewed every few years to ensure that they continue to reflect the best medical practices. Upon their adoption, they are widely distributed to all AAP members through print and Web-based media, and are available for anyone to view at http://aappolicy.aappublications.org. In short, these policy statements concisely review for everyone involved in the care of children the best of what's known about what pediatricians ought to do. That's not to say that they're infallible—there certainly can be honest disagreement among doctors reviewing the evidence, and some excellent physicians will stray from the letter of these guidelines. But all pediatricians should be familiar with their content, and should be able to discuss the rationale behind their recommendations.

Most of this book is from the point of view of an "insider," revealing the secrets that can help you get better health care for your children. In this chapter, I want to reveal information that should be known to every pediatrician, and should form the basis for many clinical decisions. One way to ensure that pediatricians have kept up with current knowledge is to see if their recommendations jibe with those of their own professional organization. If they don't, they're either maverick original thinkers—or more likely they have stopped paying attention. You should expect any good pediatrician to have an excellent working knowledge of public "uninside" information.

NUTRITION

Good nutrition starts in infancy, and there are several AAP statements concerning nursing and bottle feeding. The AAP unequivocally endorses breast feeding for all newborns, unless there is a specific medical reason why it cannot be done. Healthy newborns should be placed in skin-to-skin contact with their mothers immediately after birth until the first feeding is complete. They should not be given formula or any other fluids unless there is a specific medical reason. The AAP also recommends against pacifier use until nursing is well established. Nursing should continue for at least the first year of life, and continued beyond that for as long as the family wishes.

Although not specifically stated, the AAP seems to endorse milk-based formula over soy. Soy formulas have no advantage over milk-based products, though they're suggested for very rare babies who have hereditary syndromes that preclude milk from mammal sources, or for families who wish to adhere to a vegetarian diet. The Academy specifically recommends against the routine use of soy formulas to prevent or treat colic (fussiness), or to prevent the development of allergic diseases like food allergies, eczema, or asthma.

Babies who are exhibiting "allergic" symptoms related to their food intake can be divided into three categories:

1. *Classic, or IgE-mediated, allergy.* These symptoms include hives, wheezing, and perhaps some cases of eczema. If formula fed, the AAP recommends babies with these symptoms try a soy-based formula. Elimination of cow's milk, eggs, fish, peanuts, and tree nuts from the maternal diet is recommended for nursing babies who have these classic allergy symptoms.
2. *Enterocolitis.* These are babies with mucusy, bloody stools. If formula fed, they should be switched to a truly hypoallergenic formula like Alimentum or Nutramigen. Nursing moms should follow the restricted diet mentioned above in the rare case when allergic enterocolitis occurs in a breast-fed baby.

3. *Nonspecific possible adverse reactions.* These are babies who have fussiness, gas, or other concerns not listed above. These babies do not have true allergy, and are unlikely to benefit from expensive hypoallergenic formulas. For severe symptoms the AAP states that a one or two-week trial may be warranted.

Babies at the highest risk for developing allergic disease are those with at least two allergic first degree relatives. That is, either both parents, or a parent plus a sibling, have allergies. In this case the AAP recommends exclusive breastfeeding, with elimination of peanuts and tree nuts from mom's diet. These moms should also consider avoiding eggs, cow's milk, and fish. If formula fed, these babies at highest risk for allergy should receive one of the expensive hypoallergenic formulas. Whether nursing or bottle fed, they should have a delayed introduction to solid foods, with no solids until six months, no dairy until twelve months, no eggs until two years, and no peanuts or tree nuts until three years old.

The AAP endorses iron fortification of all infant formulas, pointing out that there is no medical reason why any baby should not receive their daily recommended iron. Iron supplementation of formula does not cause colic, gas, constipation, cramps, or any other symptoms whatsoever. In fact, the AAP recommends against the manufacture of low-iron formulas. If they are marketed, the AAP recommends that they be clearly labeled as nutritionally inadequate.

Nutritional issues for older children are also addressed in AAP statements. Juice has limited nutritional benefits, and overindulgence contributes to diarrhea, overweight (or in some "sippers," underweight), and dental cavities. Juice is not recommended until after six months of age. For children less than six years it should be limited to less than four to six ounces per day. It should not be offered in sippy cups that allow children to stroll around while sipping throughout the day.

In schools, restrictions are recommended for soft drinks, sodas, and fruit-flavored drinks. They should never be sold in competition with more nutritious food at mealtimes, and vending machines for these drinks should be eliminated entirely from elementary schools.

> ☞ **Most pediatricians do not recommend *any* juice for toddlers. It has minimal nutritional benefits and gets kids accustomed to drinking sweet beverages. To encourage the best health habits, offer only water or milk.**

Additional dietary guidelines suggested for children over two years of age include using vegetable oil or soft margarines instead of butter; eating whole-grain rather than refined grain products; using nonfat or low-fat dairy products; eating more fish; and reducing the intake of salt and processed foods.

PHYSICAL FITNESS, EXERCISE, AND TELEVISION

Sixty minutes of daily moderate to vigorous play or physical exercise is recommended by the AAP. Schools should have a comprehensive, preferably daily physical education program for children of all grades. Though strength and resistance training can safely be part of an exercise program for older kids, maximal sports like competitive weight lifting or body building should be avoided until children have completed their growth. Resistance training should be combined with aerobic training for improved overall health benefits.

Pediatricians should recognize patterns of abnormal growth, including children who are at risk of becoming overweight. The body mass index (BMI) should be calculated and plotted yearly, and pediatricians should use changes in the BMI from year to year to identify children at risk. The AAP also advocates that pediatricians treat and prevent obesity by encouraging breastfeeding, healthy eating patterns, physical activity, and unstructured play.

In policy statements the AAP refers to television, movies, videos, video games, and recreational computer use collectively as "media," and emphasizes the potential negative effects of excessive media time on children of all ages. Parents should be urged to avoid any television viewing for children less than two, and limit media time for older children to less than two hours per day. Television sets and other sources of media entertainment should not be in children's bedrooms. Reasons for limiting media exposure go beyond the amount of media time to the risks entailed by the programming itself. Exposure to media violence increases the risk of violent behavior among teens, and younger children can be traumatized by news reports about violent crimes or natural disasters. Media programming doesn't reflect an accurate or healthful portrayal of sexual relationships, and glorifies tobacco and alcohol use. The AAP endorses laws to regulate all toy-based programs in the same way traditional advertisements are regulated, decrease the amount of commercial time during children's television by 50 percent, and ban all alcohol and tobacco advertising in media.

INFANT ISSUES

Sudden Infant Death Syndrome (SIDS) is a devastating event that is still only partially understood. However, excellent studies have suggested several ways to decrease the incidence of unexpected death among young babies, and the implementation of these strategies has already eliminated about half of the SIDS deaths in the United States yearly. The AAP recommends the following steps to decrease the risk of SIDS among all babies:

- Infants should be placed on their backs to sleep. Side sleeping is not as safe and should not be recommended; sleeping a baby on the stomach is riskiest of all. Note that this is not advice to *keep* babies on their backs throughout the night; do not use any sort of wedge or other device to keep a baby from moving.
- A firm crib mattress covered with a sheet is the best sleeping surface.
- Loose or soft objects should be kept out of cribs.
- Do not smoke during pregnancy.
- A separate, but close, sleeping area for a baby is recommended. Bed-sharing increases a baby's risk of death, and cosleeping "sidecars" do not have

established safety standards. A separate crib or bassinet kept in the parent's bedroom is the safest sleeping arrangement.

- Offering a pacifier is recommended as further protection against SIDS. Pacifier use should be delayed until one month of age for nursing babies.
- Avoid overheating.
- Devices sold to reduce the risk of SIDS or as "early warning monitors" are not recommended, as they have not been shown to work.

Newborn circumcision has also attracted controversy, with some vocal advocacy groups weighing in with strong opinions. Looking at the evidence, the AAP policy is neutral on the issue. That is, while there may are some moderate health benefits (mostly a reduction in urinary tract infections among circumcised infants), they are not compelling enough to recommend that every male baby undergo this procedure. Likewise, the risks of the procedure are low enough so that the AAP feels that neonatal circumcision is ethically sound, though not medically necessary. The AAP recommends that pediatricians present a balanced view of the advantages and disadvantages of newborn circumcision, with the family making the final decision. If a decision to circumcise is made, appropriate steps should be taken to minimize pain.

INJURIES AND ACCIDENTS

Accidental injuries are the leading cause of death of children over one year of age, and the AAP has several policy statements addressing child safety issues. Some apply to infants and young children. Walkers, which have no benefits and have caused deaths, should be banned entirely; walkers already in use should be destroyed. Stationary activity centers are a safer alternative. Regarding accidental poisoning, the AAP now recommends that syrup of ipecac not be given to induce vomiting, and suggests that parents discard ipecac if they have any in their homes. Swimming programs can be fun for children of any age, but they should not be promoted to decrease the risk of drowning for infants and toddlers. Most children are not developmentally ready for formal swimming lessons until after their fourth birthday.

To prevent accidental falls, the AAP recommends several measures for people living with young children in multiple story buildings. Locks should be placed on windows to prevent them from being opened more that four inches, and operable window guards should be placed on windows on higher floors. These window guards should be moveable in case of fire. The AAP endorses legislation requiring landlords to install these devices.

Selecting and using the most appropriate vehicle safety seat for growing children can be confusing, but this should be an area of expertise for pediatricians. The AAP has specific recommendations:

- Children should face the rear of the vehicle until they are one year of age *and* weigh at least twenty pounds. For children who reach twenty pounds before their first birthday, use a convertible car seat that that can accommodate their size facing backwards.

- If the convertible car seat can accommodate children in a backwards facing position until an older age or higher weight, this position is favored for optimal protection until the child reaches a size where the car seat must face forward.
- A child should ride in the forward facing convertible safety seat with a full harness until at least forty pounds, and can continue to ride in this seat as long as it is comfortable and fits well.
- A forward-facing seat, a combination seat, or a belt-positioning booster should be used once a child has outgrown the convertible seat. A vehicle's safety belts cannot be used alone until they fit the child correctly with the shoulder belt positioned comfortably across the chest and the lap belt low and snug across the thighs. This will typically not occur until a child is over eighty pounds, though it will depend on the shape of the child and specific model of vehicle.
- For maximum safety, the AAP encourages manufacturers to develop seats that allow children to face the rear of the vehicle until they are four years old.
- Preschool children should use these same restraints on school buses.
- Traditional seat belts should be installed on all newly purchased school buses, and school systems should encourage their use.

AAP recommendations for vehicle safety go beyond cars. For bicyclists, helmets should be used during every ride. They should be replaced after any accident, or at least every five years. Children who ride as passengers should be at least one year old, wear a helmet, and ride in a secured bicycle mounted seat or better yet a bicycle-towed trailer. To improve the safety of all-terrain vehicle (ATV) use, the AAP recommends that drivers wear motorcycle helmets and that passengers not be allowed. Laws are endorsed to ban children younger than sixteen from operating ATVs and require operators to have a driver's license. The use of ATVs should be banned at night. Existing three-wheeled ATVs should be recalled, and no further three-wheeled ATVs should be sold. Although not traditionally thought of as vehicles, walk-behind lawnmowers should not be used by children less than twelve, and teenagers should be at least sixteen years old before they are allowed to operate riding mowers. Children should be at least sixteen years of age to operate personal watercraft, and any riders should always wear approved personal floatation devices.

Several specific sporting activities have received attention in AAP policy statements to make them safer. Children less than ten should be supervised during skateboard use; children less than five should not use skateboards at all. Kids younger than eight should not ride scooters without close supervision. Pediatricians are encouraged to advise skateboarders and scooter riders to wear helmets and other protective gear like wrist guards, elbow pads, and knee pads. For in-line skaters, the AAP endorses the same protective gear but goes a step further in encouraging legislation to make helmet use mandatory. Boxing is specifically opposed as a sport for any child or young adult by AAP policy.

Explosives and firearms are another source of injury. The AAP states that the most effective way to reduce firearm-related injuries is to remove guns from homes and communities through regulation, especially those that specifically ban handguns and assault weapons. Safety and design regulations are encouraged, though they are admittedly of unproven benefit. To avoid injury from fireworks, the AAP recommends that the private sale and use of fireworks be banned. Families should attend public displays rather than use fireworks on their own.

Trampoline injuries are common and potentially serious. The AAP recommends that trampolines never be used at home, either inside our outside. They should not be part of physical education programs, nor should they be installed as playground equipment. Limited use of trampolines under supervised conditions for training in certain sports may be appropriate, though in such cases several design and use recommendations are made. Among these are: a safety pad should cover all steel parts; the surface around the trampoline should be soft; ladders providing unintended access by smaller children should not be used; only one person should use a trampoline at a time, with the user at the center of the mat at all times; the trampoline should be stored securely and unreachable when not in use; and children under the age of six should be prohibited from using a trampoline at all.

MISCELLANEOUS TOPICS

Spanking can be a controversial subject, and the AAP addresses the issue from the point of view of what can be objectively proven about this disciplinary tool. Points reviewed about spanking in the AAP policy are based on solid clinical studies and research:

- It is less effective overall than time-out or removal of privileges in reducing problem behaviors.
- Although it may immediately stop an unwanted behavior, spanking becomes less effective with subsequent use.
- At best, spanking is only effective when used infrequently for selected circumstances.
- The use of spanking makes other disciplinary modes less effective. That is, once a child is spanked, it is more difficult to use time-outs or other methods effectively.
- Spanking of children less than eighteen months of age is unlikely to be of benefit because toddlers of that age will not connect their behavior to the punishment.
- The more children are hit, the more likely they are to hit their own children and spouses as adults.

The AAP has never called for a ban on spanking by parents, but the group is committed to the concept that there are more effective methods of discipline for most families that should be taught by pediatricians. The AAP has called for the banning of corporal punishment in schools.

Regarding a different issue, the AAP supports the use of generic medications if the safety and effectiveness of the generic is equivalent. In this case, the physician prescribes the medi-

> ☞ **The best reason to avoid spanking is that there are more effective ways to teach children to behave.**

cation, but the pharmacist may choose the brand that is dispensed. Different brands of generic medicines should be chemically identical. However, the AAP does not support automatically recommending generics in all situations. A related issue is "therapeutic substitution," where a pharmacist, without informing the physician, substitutes a different medication within the same category. This has been proposed on a limited scale as a cost-containment method, and is not endorsed by the AAP.

DOES YOUR PEDIATRICIAN FOLLOW THESE GUIDELINES?

AAP guidelines are not meant to be a straightjacket, and are not meant to represent the only way medicine should be practiced. But they are well researched and endorsed by the leading minds in the field of pediatrics. Pediatricians should be familiar with the information in these statements, and should have scientifically valid reasons if they give advice that contradicts the official positions of the AAP. Knowing this information is one way pediatricians should be able to demonstrate their understanding of evolving concepts in medicine.

SOURCES

All of the AAP policy statements, clinical guidelines, and supporting material are available to the general public at http://aappolicy.aappublications.org. The following is a list of the statements reviewed in this chapter, along with their years of publication. If a second year is listed, that is the year in which the academy reaffirmed their position. I urge interested parents to review these statements on their own, especially if they have heard contradicting information and wish to investigate the details behind the recommendations.

- All-terrain vehicle injury prevention: Two-, three-, and four-wheeled unlicensed motor vehicles, 2000, 2004
- Bicycle helmets, 2001
- Breastfeeding and the use of human milk, 2005
- Children, adolescents, and advertising, 1995
- Children, adolescents, and television, 2001
- Circumcision policy statement, 1999, 2005
- Corporal punishment in schools, 2000
- Dietary recommendations for children and adolescents: A guide for practitioners, 2006

- Falls from heights: Windows, roofs, and balconies, 2001, 2005
- Firearm-related injuries affecting the pediatric population, 2000, 2004
- Fireworks-related injuries in children, 2001, 2005
- Generic prescribing, generic substitution, and therapeutic substitution, 1987, 2005
- Guidance for effective discipline, 1998, 2004
- Hypoallergenic infant formulas, 2000
- Injuries associated with infant walkers, 2001
- In-line skating injuries in children and adolescents, 1998
- Iron fortification of infant formulas, 1999
- Lawnmower-related injuries in children, 2001, 2005
- Media education, 1999
- Media violence, 2001
- Participation in boxing by children, adolescents, and young adults, 1997
- Personal watercraft use by children and adolescents, 2000, 2004
- Physical fitness and activity in schools, 2000, 2004
- Poison treatment in the home, 2003
- Prevention of pediatric overweight and obesity, 2003
- School transportation safety, 1996
- Selecting and using the most appropriate car safety seats for growing children: Guidelines for counseling parents, 2002
- Soft drinks in schools, 2004
- Soy-protein based formulas: Recommendations for use in infant feeding, 1998
- Strength training by children and adolescents, 2001
- Swimming programs for infants and toddlers, 2000, 2004
- The changing concept of sudden infant death syndrome: Diagnostic coding shifts, controversies regarding the sleeping environment, and new variables to consider in reducing risk, 2005
- The use and misuse of fruit juice in pediatrics, 2001
- Trampolines at home, school, and recreation centers, 1999

4

WHAT EVERY PARENT SHOULD KNOW

The Caltermans are a colorful family. The five-year-old boy brings his complicated new toys to demonstrate for me, the three-year-old girl brings her drawings to explain to me, and the baby brings smiles and cracker crumbs to share with me. After three children, mom and I know each other very well. At the end of a visit for her third child, she said with an exhausted smile "With three kids, I'm too tired to think of any questions for you. Just tell me what I need to know." This chapter is for parents who want to know what they need to know, even if they don't know what to ask.

EAT TOGETHER

Children benefit from eating together with their families at every age. Infants learn to use utensils and drink from a cup by modeling their parents, while toddlers are more willing to try new foods if they see them being eaten by parents and siblings. Teenagers who regularly eat with their families are less likely to smoke or use alcohol or marijuana. At every age, children who eat along with their family tend to consume healthier foods, and are at less risk for becoming overweight. Mealtime is also a perfect occasion for children to practice the social skills of manners and speaking in turn. Parents benefit too; mealtime is a good opportunity to talk with your children about their day. This doesn't mean you have to eat every single meal together, but every family should make one meal a day a priority to share together. Turn off the television, sit down, and enjoy a relaxed meal together.

KEEP YOUR HANDS CLEAN

Almost all common infections are transmitted by dirty hands. The common cold, strep throat, vomiting and diarrhea viruses, pink eye—they're all infections that can be prevented by keeping your hands and your children's hands clean.

A good hand washing requires ordinary soap and water (antibacterial soaps offer no added benefit), and takes about thirty seconds. In a hurry? Use an alcohol-based hand sanitizer such as Purell. A quick squirt of sanitizer followed by a rub until your hands are dry eliminates the source of most infections, and may even be superior to hand washing.

MODEL GOOD BEHAVIOR

Babies need to learn to behave—it's not a built in ability. Most learning in younger children occurs through modeling. That is, they see what their parents do, and they try to do it. Have you ever seen a toddler walk around in circles while babbling into mom's phone? You don't need to *teach* children to talk on the phone; just model the behavior and they'll pick it up. In the same way, parents need to model appropriate social behaviors. At the dinner table, try new foods and wait your turn to speak. Don't belittle others, but offer constructive help. When you're angry, show how a mature adult handles conflict by remaining calm—or at least go somewhere else to scream. Modeling good behavior is not going to solve all of your parenting struggles, but it's an easy way to create a solid foundation for learning good behavior. Modeling doesn't end when your children are older. Set a good example to teach children of any age about how to be an adult: managing money, meeting and introducing people, respecting elders, helping handicapped people, treating animals with respect, and being a reliable friend. These and many other life lessons are better learned by example than by instruction.

TURN OFF THE TELEVISION

When you include all video-based entertainment, children in the United States spend an average of six and a half hours a day, seven days a week, in front of a screen. That's more time than they spend in school, and second only to sleep in time spent on daily activities.

Children who watch more television are more likely to be overweight, and more likely to do poorly in school. Their diet tends to include more fatty processed foods, and they get less exercise. Not only is TV watching entirely sedentary, it also exposes children to harmful messages about health and their bodies. Look at what the food and restaurant commercials are promoting—huge portions of processed junk. Look at the shapes of the models, especially women—is there any wonder why so many teenage girls are preoccupied with their waistlines? The shows themselves are loaded with commercial messages encouraging unhealthy consumerism along with powerful violent and sexual images. Kids should not be expected to handle the sort of material that we've accepted as ordinary TV entertainment.

There are ways to make TV watching more healthful for children. Limit the amount of time spent with the television on, and limit TV to prerecorded material that you know has appropriate content for your child's age. Watch

TV as a family so that you can discuss the shows together. Keep televisions out of kids' bedrooms. A limited amount of television can be a relaxing and entertaining time for a family, but you need to prevent this from getting out of hand.

Keep Track of Your Child's Medical Information

The world of health care delivery is complex. Many patients rely on multiple doctors and pharmacies, and get tests done at multiple places. Although you'd expect your pediatric office to be the one place where all records are kept, sometimes this system doesn't work as well as it should. If your child's allergist orders some blood tests, your pediatrician might never get a copy of those results; likewise, records from emergency room visits may not ever become part of your child's chart. Think of your pediatrician's records as the best repository of all information, but remember that some items might not get there without your help. Request copies of all test results, all consultant letters, and all lab reports; give these to your pediatrician after making a copy for yourself. Keep copies for yourself and your pediatrician of any after-hours visits, or any health care encounters that take place out of town. You should also keep your own copy of all immunization records, and be sure your pediatrician's copy of this information is accurate. A complete and accessible medical record can be a crucial resource if your child ever becomes seriously ill.

Your Family Is More Important than Your Child

Your child is precious, but don't lose sight of your overall family's health. For example, I've seen marriages dissolve over problems at bedtime, where children refuse to sleep in their own beds. Though fixing this problem is challenging, it is wrong to sacrifice a marriage over a child's sleep preferences. (I'm not saying it's wrong for a child to share a bed if that's what both parents want to do, but rather that the health of the parents and their marriage should not be sacrificed in a case where the parents need their bed for themselves.) In another example, one child might refuse to eat what's served, disrupting the family's meals. Rather than giving up on having family meals altogether, the child who is the problem can be excluded from the meal until improved habits are learned. Even better, he or she could be allowed to participate in the social setting of the meal even if nothing is actually eaten. The bottom line is that a healthy child requires a healthy family, and you should not sacrifice your family's health over any problems one of your children might be having.

Drive Safely

Motor vehicle accidents are the leading cause of death for children. Be as safe as possible: use age-appropriate restraints correctly, and avoid distractions like cellular phone calls and fiddling with the radio. It might be tempting to use a small mirror to spy on your children, but it's an unacceptable distraction.

Don't drive when you're on sedating medications or alcohol, or even when you're tired. Try not to go out if the weather is unsafe, and obey the speed limit. These simple measures could save thousands of children's lives each year.

SOME DOCTORS ARE QUACKS

Beware. Though we're all trained and licensed, many doctors are out there practicing bad medicine. Some are following outdated ideas by not keeping up on recent advances in therapeutics and science. Others have grown lazy, and are quick to prescribe antibiotics for what we know are viral infections. A few take advantage of trusting patients by selling overpriced cosmetics or administering worthless vitamin injections. Every doctor knows a few colleagues that have crossed the line, and are no longer responsible physicians. Unfortunately, state medical boards are reluctant to take action against lousy doctors unless truly egregious mistakes are proven. If you're starting to wonder whether your pediatrician is not consistently practicing good medicine, look for a second opinion to review your child's health care plan.

WITH NUTRITION, IT'S THE BIG PICTURE THAT MATTERS

In many ways, traditional nutrition advice is misleading. "Eat balanced meals" doesn't really make sense. It's your child's overall intake that determines if the diet is healthy; it doesn't matter one bit if any individual meal is balanced. "Take your vitamins" is lousy advice for most kids too. After all, almost all grains and dairy products are fortified with vitamins and minerals, and vitamin deficiencies have become very rare in the United States and other developed countries.

Clearly, though, the diet of children needs to be improved. There has been a dramatic rise in obesity among children, parallel to the increase seen in adults. In the United States, about one in three children is overweight—with a predictable increase seen in related health consequences like diabetes, joint problems, and cardiovascular disease. Many children are relying on processed foods, refined sugars, soft drinks, and fast-food restaurants as their primary sources of nutrition.

A diet that relies on whole grains, fresh produce, and home-cooked meals dramatically decreases the risk of overweight and diabetes. The best nutrition advice that your pediatrician ought to be telling you is to limit portions, cut out processed foods, and eat as a family at home.

YOU CAN GET GOOD MEDICINE WITHOUT MEDICATION

By good medicine, I mean the steps you need to take to keep your children healthy. In many cases, no medicine is required at all. Children who are having trouble in school might need a better night's sleep or a pair of eyeglasses; children who have a sore throat might benefit more from a milkshake than from any medication or antibiotic. That isn't to say that medication isn't an important tool for any pediatrician, it's just that it should not be the only approach taken to health problems. Too often, pediatricians and parents feel that a doctor's visit is wasted time if the parent doesn't leave with a prescription for medication. Keep in mind that all medications have side effects—they're potent biologic agents, and if they have any possible benefit then there must be a potential for adverse reactions. The only medicines that could possibly be 100 percent safe are those that are entirely placebos (see Chapter 11). As a parent, you should be wary of any physician who too quickly reaches for the prescription pad.

5

GET THE MOST OUT
OF EVERY DOCTOR VISIT

Have you ever seen a busy pediatrician's schedule? If you've found a good doctor, you can bet other families have found that office, too. The schedules are tight, and there's a limited amount of time to get your answers. Armed with insider knowledge, you'll be able to get what you need out of every visit, without feeling rushed.

There are several different types of appointments: ordinary sick visits, well checks, follow-ups, or other variations on these basics. Before discussing the details of these visit types, I want to stress the most important rule for getting the most out of any visit: focus. Though there are different types of doctor visits for different problems, the key to getting the most out of any doctor visit is to keep the family and the doctor focused on the main problem.

FOR ANY VISIT: FOCUS

In a typical office, a nurse or assistant will first bring your family back to an exam room. The nurse will probably measure vital signs and the child's weight, and ask why you came. State in a few brief words exactly why you came to the doctor, and say your main concern first. For a young child, this conversation is with a parent, but I always prefer for older kids to speak for themselves. When the doctor arrives, the family should reiterate their main worry. Medical people call this a "chief complaint," and it helps focus everyone's attention for the visit.

Good, well-spoken chief complaints are simple and to the point:

- "Joe's cough is keeping him awake."
- "Maggie has an itchy rash."
- "Victoria is struggling in school."

Meandering, wandering, or misleading chief complaints will do neither you nor the doctor any good:

- "Well, John's headaches are getting better, I think they were from allergies. I took him off his medicine. But today at school he had a fever."
- "Olivia has had diarrhea for a long time. And her stomach hurts. Today she fell and hurt her wrist. Well, the diarrhea seems better now."

If you've seen the same doctor before for a similar issue, drop in a reminder of something specific that will jog the doctor's memory:

- "Last time my asthma acted up because my mom visited with her smoking boyfriend."

If you've seen someone else in the group for the same problem, remind the doctor so the old record can be reviewed:

- "In March we saw Dr. Jernigan for Casey's belly aches."

After listening to your chief complaint, the doctor will ask several questions in order to obtain the "history of present illness." These questions usually relate to the timing and causes of symptoms. Feel free to elaborate on details that you think the doctor needs to know, but resist the temptation to start bringing up unrelated information. Again, the idea is to focus on your main concern first.

You can bring up other issues after your discussion of the main issue. If there are just a few minor things, you should ask the doctor to address them at the same visit. You'll want to bring up secondary concerns before the physical exam starts, so the doctor knows what to look for. If you have several elaborate problems, it is best to ask if the doctor would rather address everything in one visit or would prefer for you to schedule another appointment.

> ☞ **If you try to get every single possible problem on a long laundry list addressed in one encounter, you are more likely to get superficial answers.**

During the physical exam, the discussion of the history can continue, and the physician may begin to discuss the diagnosis and treatments. Try not to speak when we have a stethoscope in our ears; it's distracting, and we can't hear you anyway!

If you have a struggling toddler or baby, ask the physician for the best way you can help. There are times for discussing cooperation with the child, and times for little bribes, and times for just holding them still. Every pediatrician has a few tricks to help with distraction, and a few backup tricks to help hold children still as safely as possible to get a good exam without causing more trauma.

The doctor will then complete the physical exam and discuss the likely diagnosis and treatment options. Now is the time to ask questions and voice any misgivings. It does no one any good if a family leaves quietly disappointed—speak up if you are not satisfied.

A well child visit can include all of the above, and the doctor can certainly address some "sick" issues at the same time. But remember at a well visit the doctor will try to go through a lot of information on diet, growth, and development; the physical exam should be much more comprehensive; and the physician will want to discuss some points of "anticipatory guidance". These are tips and suggestions for what challenges to expect for your child's age. Because there is so much material to go over in a comprehensive well child visit, it is difficult to have the time to add an elaborate discussion of a complex health problem. Ask the physician if the well check is the best time to go into an involved sick complaint.

When the Wrong Focus Can Be Misleading

Focus on the *symptoms* that are most concerning to you at your visits, but try not to use a *diagnosis* as your chief complaint. Jumping to a specific diagnosis too early can lead the doctor and patient along the wrong path.

A new patient came to see me for the first time, Eduardo. At sixteen, he did most of the talking. His chief complaint was: "You've got to help me with my sinus headaches." He told me about his multiple visits to allergists and sinus specialists because of years of sinus headaches and misery. When I asked him to just describe his symptoms, it became clear to me that his headaches were very typical of migraine, and not in any way suggestive of sinus pressure headaches. With a short discussion of prevention techniques for migraines, Eduardo was able to almost completely eliminate his headaches.

At some point, Eduardo or one of his many doctors had declared these headaches as "sinus." Only by trying to take that diagnosis off the table and discuss the symptoms was I able to get to the true diagnosis. The lesson here is to use your main *symptom* as a chief complaint, not your suspected diagnosis.

Remember, the key to any successful doctor visit is clear communication: what exact problems am I trying to get addressed and what exactly is the doctor telling me to do? Try your best to be clear in bringing up concerns and answering questions, and expect physicians to be clear about how they suggest you proceed.

THE SICK VISIT

Pediatrician visits come in many types, but the two most common are well and sick. Though some of the components overlap, their goals are different. A sick visit should be entirely driven by the concerns of the family, while a well visit should be at least partially driven by what the doctor thinks needs to be reviewed for that age group. In this section we'll go through the elements of a sick visit, and illustrate how a doctor arrives at a diagnosis and treatment plan. I'll also go through the doctor lingo that describes each part of the encounter so you understand what's going on from inside the white coat.

The typical sick encounter with a pediatrician goes like this:

1. Vital signs are recorded while a nurse takes a brief history.
2. The patient or parent tells the doctor what the problem is (the "chief complaint").
3. The doctor asks for details (this is the "history of present illness").
4. A physical exam is performed.
5. The diagnosis is discussed.
6. Plans are made for treatment and follow-up.

Other things might take place too, including a review of prior illnesses or family history. Sometimes, labs and x-rays will be done. But the general outline for a sick encounter is the same: talk, examine, and then make plans. One time-honored way for physicians to organize encounters in this fashion is the so-called "SOAP format," where SOAP is an acronym for:

Subjective (the chief complaint and other history, the talking part)
Objective (the physical exam, and any lab or other "hard" data)
Assessment (the diagnosis)
Plan

Next we'll go through the elements of the a visit and show you how the doctor uses each of them to arrive at a plan, and how you can help make sure that the doctor makes the best possible decisions.

Chief Complaint

In most situations, the nurse brings back the family and asks something like "What are you here for today?" This is the time to be direct and to the point. Say in as few words possible exactly what you're worried about. Once this is written down it focuses the entire visit on that issue. If you have several issues you wish to have addressed, *start with the one that is most important to you.* This is phenomenally important, as you do not want to doctor to spend most of the time reviewing secondary problems.

Vital Signs

After recording the chief complaint, the nurse or assistant will usually record appropriate vital signs. Keep in mind that many vital signs have a normal range that varies with the age of your child, so don't assume that a blood pressure that sounds normal for an adult is normal for a child. Although not every one of these is necessary at every visit, the customary vital signs are:

- *Temperature:* Measuring and recording the temperature is traditionally part of most sick visits, though if you bring your child in to discuss a twisted ankle I'm not sure a thermometer is necessary. If you've recorded your child's temperature at home, tell the nurses what the number on the thermometer was and how you recorded it. Don't add a degree or in any way "adjust" the measurement; just tell us what the number was. That's the clearest way to communicate what was measured.
- *Heart rate:* Both the heart rate and rhythm should be recorded. Higher heart rates are not generally a good thing, unless the child was just exercising. An elevated heart rate can be a sign of dehydration, fear, fever, heart failure, or certain medicines. A low heart rate in pediatrics is most often seen in a well-trained athlete, but can indicate a serious problem with the heart's rhythm. Once in a while an irregular heart beat can be heard. This may be normal if it is an occasional "extra beat" or if the heart rate clearly varies as the child breathes in and out.
- *Blood pressure:* Because it is difficult to measure blood pressure in younger kids, in pediatrics this is routinely checked only at well visits for children older than 3 or so. Blood pressure should also be determined during the evaluation of certain medical problems, such as headaches, puffy extremities or eyes, or blood in the urine. If a young child is scared and screaming, it is better to write down "unable to record blood pressure because of screaming" than to write down an inaccurate figure.
- *Respiratory rate:* This is a very important vital sign in pediatrics. A normal respiratory rate virtually guarantees the lungs are healthy, no matter how much the child is coughing. But rapid breathing in a child means one of only a few things: the child has a fever, or has significant lung, heart, or metabolic disease.
- *Weight:* I count this as a vital sign, as important as the others. Pediatricians need an accurate weight to dose medicines, but also to see how a child is doing overall. In the short run, say over a few days, weight loss always means dehydration. A longer term problem with weight, either a weight loss or a failure to gain weight as expected, may be an important sign of serious illness or feeding problems.
- *Height:* The height is important, but can be difficult to measure accurately in a squirming toddler. Failure to gain height as expected should always prompt a thorough investigation.

More about Measuring Temperatures

What's the best way to measure a child's temperature? Believe it or not, there's disagreement on this basic question even among pediatricians. Keep in mind that if your child doesn't feel warm, you probably don't need to measure a temperature. Parents are very good at telling if their own baby has a fever, though neither parents nor health care professionals are very good at estimating the magnitude of a fever by touch alone.

There are many types of thermometers:

- *Rectal:* The only acceptable way to measure the temperature in babies less than three months is a rectal thermometer. In those very young babies, knowing the exact rectal temperature is necessary to make the best decisions about what evaluation is necessary. For children older than a year, don't measure temperatures rectally. It's accurate, but unpleasant and unnecessary. Rectal, oral, and axillary thermometers can all be made of traditional glass, or can be digital. The digital ones are the best to use in all circumstances—they're quicker and safer.
- *Ear:* "Tympanic membrane" thermometers are terrible. They're difficult to use and inaccurate even in the hands of trained nurses.
- *Temporal artery:* These thermometers use a little probe that is rubbed across the forehead in one swoop. They're accurate, easy, fast, and not too expensive. Many children's hospitals are starting to rely on these for children past the newborn period.
- *Oral:* They were good enough for grandma, and oral thermometers still work fine. The inexpensive glass ones take a few minutes to get a reading. Don't put thermometers that use mercury in anyone's mouth. For an oral thermometer, the column should be red, which is a safe chemical, rather than silver mercury. Better yet, choose a quicker digital model.
- *Axillary:* I call these "chicken wing" temperatures; use an oral thermometer and hold it under your child's "wing" until it beeps. They take too long, and kids often squirm away before an accurate reading is reached.

The winner? For children older than three months, get a temporal artery thermometer. Babies younger than this, unfortunately, have to be checked the old fashioned way!

HISTORY OF PRESENT ILLNESS

This part of the visit is usually performed by the physician. We'll want to know the details of how the concerns arose:

- When did it start?
- How does it vary from day to day—is it constant or intermittent?
- What makes it better? What makes it worse?
- What treatments have you tried?
- Has it ever happened before?
- What else is going on, or what other symptoms are there?

Open-ended questions might be followed by more specific questions about the quality and nature of the symptom, or exposures from the environment or other people that might be contributing to the problem.

At the end of the history of present illness, the physician will usually know the diagnosis, or at least have a short list of possibilities in mind. The remainder of the visit is to confirm that impression and flesh out the best way to address it.

Review of Systems

In a review of systems, the doctor will ask about other items that might be going on. If the patient hasn't already mentioned these things, the doctor will often ask questions about the presence of common symptoms like:

- Fever
- Cough
- Runny nose
- Belly aches
- Vomiting or diarrhea
- Rash
- Many others, depending on the chief complaint

Many doctors, myself included, sort of fold the review of systems into the history, asking questions about both issues interchangeably. But technically the history of present illness is for the patient to talk about the thing that made them come to the doctor, and the review of systems is for the doctor to ask about anything else.

Other History

Depending on the nature of the problem, other history items might be important to help diagnose and treat the problem:

- *Social history:* Who does the child live with? How is the family getting along? How is school?
- *Family history:* What illnesses run in the family?
- *Past medical history:* What problems have there been in the past?
- *Birth history:* This is pediatrics. Sometimes we want to start from the beginning!

The Physical Exam

It's magical, it's personal, and it involves touching. I am amazed and honored that kids let us get away with doing this! Not only can I learn some important things from a physical exam, but it is also an essential way to build trust and a therapeutic relationship between a child and physician.

Every physician has a different way of doing a physical exam, including a different order and different techniques for distraction. Certainly the exam should focus on areas of concern, but should also include important related areas. Some general points that should be true of any exam:

- It should not be rushed.
- The child should be calm and quiet, as much as possible. I'll go through just about any contortion, sitting on the floor or even taking the whole family outside, if it helps the child relax enough to get a good exam.
- It isn't just for show—the physician needs to concentrate. Some conversation is OK, but there is no way to really hear what parents are saying once the stethoscope is in the ears.
- The exam should respect the privacy of the child. Some sense of decorum and privacy will develop in most children by age four, but at any age the patient should be treated with respect.
- During the exam, the child and doctor should talk about what's going on. I like to tell the kids what I need to do next. At some ages, it is fun to let the child try out some of the equipment, looking in my ears for monkeys before I get a turn.

The Assessment

So, Doc, what is going on? Now's the time for the physician to tell you what the diagnosis is, or at least a short list of what the diagnosis might be. If your pediatrician talks in mumbo-jumbo fancy doctor words, ask for a clarification. Have the doctor write down the diagnosis for your further research later.

For some problems there might not yet be a specific diagnosis. Or maybe the physician is reluctant to discuss the specifics in front of the child. A careful, astute physician may not always desire to name a diagnosis, and may in some cases just reiterate the chief complaint without specific clarification:

- "I can tell these belly aches are causing you problems, let's talk about how you can start to feel better."
- "You're discouraged that school isn't going so well. Mom, we need to talk about this some more."

Even without a specific diagnosis, by this point of the visit you should know what the doctor thinks is the problem.

The Plan

The plan should be discussed and reviewed, and the doctor needs to make sure that the family understands what is being suggested. There are three kinds of plans:

- A *diagnostic plan* is optional—when the diagnosis is clear, no further tests are needed. At other times x-rays, blood tests, or referrals are needed. Often the physician will have a nurse go over exactly what you're supposed to do to get tests accomplished.

- There should always be a *therapeutic plan*, how to begin to address the problem. Even before the tests are back (if any), some discussion of symptom relief and what to do next needs to occur.
- The *follow-up plan* is very important. It may include another visit to the doctor, or a statement like "Call us in a week if you are not better." Make sure you understand how quickly to expect to recover, and when to contact the physician if things are not going well.

Not every element occurs in every sick visit, and the length of time required for a thorough sick visit depends on the type of problem, its severity, and how it is affecting the family. But every sick visit should begin with clear communication from the family: "This is why we're here." And every sick visit should end with clear instructions from the physician suggesting what to do about it.

> **Before you leave, you should know what the doctor expects you to do.**

THE WELL VISIT

Regular routine well child visits are a great way to keep your child healthy. You should learn about the problems and challenges expected at your child's age, and how to deal with them before they become serious issues. You'll also have a chance to ask about specific concerns, and follow up on ongoing issues.

There are unique advantages to well visits:

- Your child's growth will be systematically measured and charted. Normal growth is very reassuring. But if there is a problem with your child's growth, it is far better to identify and address it early.
- You and the doctor can go through every ongoing health issue to update progress and concerns. This can be especially helpful for issues like asthma, allergies, or trouble in school.
- Well visits provide an opportunity for developmental screening at regular set intervals.
- Immunizations can be reviewed and kept up to date.
- Health screening issues can be addressed (for example, screening questionnaires can look for risk of lead exposure, tuberculosis risk, or family troubles).
- Regular well visits give families an opportunity to become comfortable and familiar with their pediatrician. Children who already know and trust their doctor will fare much better if serious illness ever strikes.
- Though there will be time to address the parents' concerns, the well visit is the best time for pediatricians to follow our own agenda, giving advice that is appropriate for your child's age. Pediatricians who have gotten to know your family will guide you along issues that are most relevant for you.

Timing of Well Child Visits

Well visits occur more frequently when your baby is younger, because growth and other issues need to be watched more closely. It is also difficult to ensure that the doctor will always get a good exam—babies cry sometimes—so it makes sense to repeat the visits regularly. Although the exact timing varies, at my office we recommend well child visits at two weeks, one month, two months, four months, six months, nine months, twelve months, fifteen months, eighteen months, two years, two and a half years, three years, and yearly thereafter. In the preteen school age kids (say from five to twelve years) every other year well checks are fine as long as the child has few ongoing issues. Teenagers often have so many things going on that even yearly visits seem inadequate!

Don't Turn Your Well Visit into a Sick Visit

Though at each well visit you'll have an opportunity to address some problems that might be on your mind, resist the temptation to "save up" all of your problems for the next checkup. If you and your physician spend most of the time of the well visit concentrating on specific concerns, you'll miss the important overall goal of the well visit: to systematically review all aspects of your child's health, and provide guidance for the challenges that are likely to occur at your child's specific age.

Unique Parts of the Well Visit

We've already reviewed many of the things that are part of a sick visit, including the chief complaint, history, physical exam, assessment, and plan. All of these are also included in the well visit, plus some other unique items.

Expanded vital signs should be measured. At each well visit, in addition to routine vitals your child should have their pulse recorded. Blood pressure is also added once a child is three years old.

Growth parameters should be carefully measured: weight at every visit; length and head circumference for children less than three, height for older than three. (Length and height are not the same thing. Length is lying down, height is standing up. For children at an age where they can do either, the height is up to $\frac{1}{2}$ inch shorter than the length. To keep measurements standard and comparable, length is the preferred way to measure children until age three.) In addition, most practices rely on the calculated body mass index (BMI) to get an overall picture of a child's potential problems with underweight or overweight. The BMI should be plotted from year to year starting at age three. Not only should all of these numbers be carefully and accurately recorded at each well visit, but your doctor should go over them with you. Ideally the office should give you a copy of all of these numbers as well, so you can keep track of them yourselves. They're fun to put in the baby book.

Old or ongoing problems should be reviewed. I like to go over every past problem to see if it is still an issue. I'd also like to hear a recap of any visits to specialists, or any medical care that occurred outside of my office.

- "I see we discussed headaches last fall—is that still a problem?"
- "Last year you were worried that your kids fight too much—how are they getting along now?"
- "I remember we sent you to an orthopedist for his elbow pain, how did that work out?"
- "Have you been to any emergency rooms or urgent care centers since our last visit?"

A comprehensive physical exam should be performed. For an ordinary sick visit, it is entirely fair for the doctor to concentrate on the area of concern, rather than do a full physical. For instance, if your child hurts his arm, the doctor is not obligated to look at his ears—though he may do so, especially if he knows your child is prone to ear infections. Some parts of the exam are traditionally neglected until a well visit, including exams of the genitals, skin, back, and nervous system. Usually, a comprehensive well exam on an older child includes a "sports fitness" exam of the major joints, muscles, and bones.

Anticipatory guidance is an essential part of every well visit. This term refers to age-specific advice about your child. The advice is meant to review problems that are likely to come up, not necessarily problems that have already begun. Believe me, issues are much easier to deal with if you've already heard about them from your doctor—you're more confident, and you know that what is going on is not unexpected. Issues that can be covered in anticipatory guidance might depend on your child's age, the time of year, and current items on the news. They'll also depend on the expertise and interests of your doctor. Some examples:

- *Appropriate toys for age:* Four month olds are getting bored with the bouncy seat. It's time for an exercise saucer.
- *Discipline:* Expect your eighteen-month-old child to start having tantrums soon; let's talk about how to handle them.
- *Eating issues:* Expect your two-year-old to have a decreasing appetite. Offer smaller portions so he doesn't just pick out his favorites.
- *Family and marital advice:* Now that your baby is a few months old, her parents need to have some time on their own.
- *Health issues:* Use mosquito repellent and sunscreen in the summer.
- *Healthy lifestyle advice:* Less television time correlates with less obesity.
- *Household issues:* Check your smoke detectors.
- *Safety:* Wear a bike helmet.
- *Sibling problems:* Don't try to micromanage their conflicts.

Immunizations will be part of many well checks, especially for children in the first two years of life. These are a very important part of keeping your child healthy, and are the most rigorously studied substances ever put into a human body. As more evidence accumulates, their safety is becoming more and more assured. There are both routine immunizations as well as other vaccines suggested for certain individuals (for example, travelers or those with special health problems). Your pediatrician should be able to discuss all of these with you.

Screening tests may be routinely suggested at certain ages. These may include screening for iron deficiency, vision problems, hearing issues, or other items. Keep in mind that most of these tests done at well child visits are "screening exams", with a high number of "false positives." If your child fails the screen, it means a more in-depth evaluation is warranted, but that does not always mean that there really is a problem. See Chapter 13 for more information about the purpose and limitations of screening tests.

Common Screening Tests and Controversies

You might think that screening procedures performed at the doctors office are all standardized, and that most physicians agree on exactly what should be done, and when. It turns out that there is quite a bit of controversy about some of these tests:

Developmental screening. Although almost all pediatricians use a series of informal brief questions to screen for developmental delay, some pediatricians have begun to rely on formal standardized checklists. Parents are typically asked to fill these out in advance or in the waiting room. There are legitimate concerns that these in-depth checklists may only increase anxiety by identifying borderline children who may not need therapy. The United States Preventative Services Task Force found in 2006 that there was insufficient evidence to recommend for or against the routine use of these screening checklists.

Hearing. Most states now mandate that newborns have their hearing screened before they leave the hospital, which takes pediatric offices "off the hook." Still, hearing problems can arise later. Fortunately it is fairly simple to reliably test hearing in a child at age four. If your child is younger than four and needs a hearing test, you should be referred to an audiologist. There has been a surge in hearing loss among teenagers related to loud music, especially when enjoyed through headphones; some pediatric practices are adding a hearing screen during the teen years to look for this.

Iron check. Iron deficiency anemia is the most common micronutrient deficiency in the developed world, and can lead to developmental and cognitive delays. The problem is that there is no simple, reliable test commonly available to detect all cases. The common finger-prick measurement of hemoglobin performed at many offices will miss many cases of iron deficiency. Some experts suggest we should have all young children take iron supplements rather than even try to find out which ones are iron-deficient.

Urinalysis. It's cheap, easy, and painless, but economic studies have failed to show that routinely performing urinalyses at well visits will really find enough genuine problems to justify the expense. The American Academy of Pediatrics suggests performing a urinalysis only twice during a youngster's life unless there are specific reasons to do them more frequently.

Vision. It is difficult to measure vision when children are younger than four years without special equipment and training. But by that age, significant problems with vision may become difficult to treat. Poor vision in a child needs to be identified as young as possible, ideally well before school entry. Though some pediatricians use special equipment to screen vision at a very young age, the insurance reimbursement for these tests is poor or nonexistent. Pediatric offices are forced to buy expensive equipment that adds to their overhead if they want to do the best job in screening for vision problems.

Don't forget your forms at home. Many children will need forms signed for camp, school, sports, or daycare. Some states have standard forms for immunizations, but bring whatever you need to have filled out and signed. Personally, I don't mind if parents fill out parts of the form if they know the answers. That saves me time.

Insiders know that a good well visit can not only include a comprehensive review of your child's health and progress, but can also provide important guidance to help keep your child happy, healthy, and safe. If you're not getting this kind of service at your pediatrician's office, now you know that you can expect more.

THE FOLLOW-UP VISIT

We've already reviewed what goes on at typical well and sick visits, and the best ways for you to make the most out of these common appointments. There is a third common kind of appointment in a pediatric office, which is underused and underappreciated: the follow-up visit.

Unlike our adult medicine colleagues, pediatricians are not especially geared toward the management of chronic problems. Doctors who serve adults see far more chronic illness: hypertension, adult diabetes, congestive heart failure, and all of the diseases associated with aging, smoking, and obesity. But a pediatrician can be an excellent resource for our patients' chronic illnesses too:

asthma, eczema, allergies, abdominal pain, headaches, school problems, recurring ear infections, obesity, chronic constipation, and many other complaints that are common in children. These problems are best addressed with regular input from a pediatrician rather than visits during the occasional crisis.

A follow-up visit is meant to revisit an issue that has already been diagnosed *in that office*. This means if your child is diagnosed with pneumonia at a local hospital emergency room and needs to be rechecked, that recheck with your doctor is NOT a follow-up. Your doctor, having never seen this problem before in your child, will have to start from the beginning and review all of the information from the outside facility—this is not what a follow-up is for. A follow-up visit starts with "how are you doing with this problem since your last visit here", rather than "tell me about how this problem started." Your doctor's office will assume that if you've made a follow-up appointment the doctor already knows what has happened before, and just needs to catch up on new developments.

> ☞ **The goal of treating any chronic health problem is to keep the child well, not just fix them every time they get sick.**

Ideally, follow-up visits should be scheduled with the physician who diagnosed the problem in the first place; but scheduling issues may force you to see a partner in the office. In that case the records will be easily accessible and can be reviewed, even though you'll be seeing a different doctor. For ongoing, chronic problems, you should see the same doctor each time. If you want a new opinion, schedule a visit with a different doctor as a sick encounter. The new physician will likely have an extensive history that will take time to review.

Most follow-up visits should be for one of two reasons: either a single visit to ensure that a one-time diagnosis has resolved, or as an ongoing regular visit to review a chronic health issue.

One-time follow-ups are common for problems such as pneumonia or other serious infections, surgical issues (though these are usually seen by the surgeon), or after any hospitalization. Most pediatricians encourage follow-up visits to recheck ears after treatment for an ear infection, which can be helpful for younger kids who cannot clearly verbalize symptoms or kids who have had problems with many ear infections.

Insiders know that follow-up visits are *not* necessary for older kids with routine ear infections, or after an ordinary strep throat. These kinds of visits are big moneymakers in some pediatric practices and are of no help to the patients.

Tips to help take advantage of follow-up visits:

- *Use them.* Especially if your child has a chronic health issue, do not wait to see the doctor only when your child is ill. Regular scheduled follow-ups during periods of wellness can help reinforce good maintenance habits to keep your child healthy. Remember that your child doesn't have to be sick to see the doctor, and a good doctor would rather concentrate on keeping your child well than merely stamping out the flames every time there is a problem.

- *Be prepared.* Bring lists of medicines your child is taking, or better yet bring a baggy of the medicine bottles themselves. You'd be surprised how often I discover a mistake in how a medicine is used if I can actually pick up the bottle and review it with the family.
- *Be honest.* What is your child taking, really? If you haven't been taking a medicine as prescribed, tell the doctor. She'll be in a better position to judge what's going on if she knows the true picture.
- *Be thorough.* If you've seen specialists about the same problem, bring any labs or x-rays or other things they have ordered, and bring any medicines they have prescribed. Depending on the problem, it can be very helpful to bring a symptom diary, showing how your child is doing from day to day and what factors might be leading to flare-ups.
- *Be assertive, but reasonable in your expectations.* Even if your doctor can't prevent all symptoms, she can at least explain what you can expect within the limitations of the best therapy.

Children have many problems that can be best addressed through regular follow-up with your pediatrician. Though these visits are usually short and focused on a single issue, they are an ideal opportunity to ensure that problems are solved, or at least managed in the best way.

OTHER TYPES OF VISITS

Not all offices offer these, but you might run into some other visit types.

Consultation

This is a visit between parents and the pediatrician, with no children present (at least no children old enough to pay attention). At consult visits behavioral or social issues that might be difficult to discuss in front of a child are reviewed. These visits can also be very valuable to calmly discuss behavioral issues with young children—if they're tearing apart the exam room, it's difficult for anyone to pay attention.

Phone Consultation

These can be very helpful for certain delicate situations, or if parents are out of town, or if it is difficult to get both parents together to review an important problem. Phone calls do create some difficulties with communication. It is harder to read emotions and body language over the phone, and it can be harder to act as a "referee" when multiple family members have different viewpoints. Also, there are practical matters of reimbursement, as most insurance companies will not pay for telephone-only visits.

Weight Checks

I discourage informal weight checks for newborns. The problem is that once the weight is measured the parents of newborns still need someone to tell them whether that weight is adequate. If it is not, someone has to figure out why. Parents should bring their newborns in for a check a few days after leaving the hospital, with a scheduled appointment to see the doctor. That way we can review not only the weight but also family issues, the baby's color and stool patterns, mom's health, and any other concerns that have come up.

Get to know what visit types your pediatrician offers, so you can request the correct type of appointment. When in doubt, ask. Whether a well, sick, follow-up, or any other kind of visit, keep your focus on your main concern to take the best advantage of your pediatrician's time and skills. Although you can't expect a single visit to solve all of your problems, you should feel that you have plan for diagnosis and treatment at the end of every encounter with your pediatrician.

6

Telephone Etiquette: When and How to Call the Doctor after Hours

I chose to practice pediatrics. In fact, every pediatrician chose to go into this field. We knew what we were getting into. Kids get sick, and kids have bad timing. Sometimes they get sick in the middle of the night or on weekends at Disneyworld. So pediatricians expect phone calls. Calling back anxious parents is part of our job.

Conscientious parents want to learn how to *know* when they ought to call. What's an emergency? What can wait until business hours? And pediatricians would really like to have the best of both worlds: we *want* to be called, without hesitation, for situations that genuinely need our input. The real emergencies, the decisions that are best made by your own doctor: these are calls that we need to get. But we like a good night's sleep as much as anyone, and some calls, shall we say, we could do without.

In this chapter I'll go over some important rules: when to call and when not to call. I'll review the sort of information you ought to have available before your call, so your doctor can make the best decisions. And I'll review some of the most common reasons for after-hours phone calls, and some good ways for parents to take the initial care steps on their own. You should not hesitate to call your pediatrician when you are genuinely worried. With the insider tips from this chapter, you'll be more confident and prepared to get your pediatrician awake when you should.

The Rules in Brief

For quick reference, the rules for when to have your doctor paged after hours are presented here first. I'll then go over them in more detail. Note that these are meant as general guidelines or suggestions. If you're worried for a reason that isn't on the list, go ahead and call.

When to call (or, "When it can't wait"):

- Trouble breathing
- Dehydration

- Acting really ill
- In unbearable pain
- When parents are really worried
- Anything involving a newborn

When not to call (or, "When it can wait until morning")

- Any administrative or insurance matter
- Routine refills
- Any long-term problem that's stable

The Rules Explained

Call When Your Child Is Having Trouble Breathing

Babies who are having trouble breathing will breathe quickly. To look for other signs of trouble, take off their shirt, and see if you can see their ribs with every breath. Look to see if their little heads are bobbing up and down with each breath, or if their nostrils are flaring. For older kids, one of the best ways to know if a child is really having trouble breathing is if they can't complete a sentence normally. Any child who has to pause between every few words for a breath is having significant difficulty. Noisy breathing might just be from a lot of nasal congestion, but if accompanied by these other symptoms it means trouble. Any child who appears to be bluish needs *immediate* medical attention.

If your child is gasping, bluish, or unable to speak or cough, call 911 *first.* Do not hesitate. For the more mild signs of respiratory distress listed above, call your pediatrician.

Call If Your Child Is Becoming Dehydrated

Vomiting, diarrhea, or fever can all lead to dehydration, and combinations of two or three of these together are even more likely to land your child in trouble. If despite these symptoms your child continues to takes sips of appropriate fluids, you're unlikely to end up with a seriously dehydrated kid. But children who are feeling ill and refusing to sip can quickly get dehydrated if they're losing fluids. Signs of dehydration include dry or tacky mouths and lips, a rapid heartbeat, cool extremities, and decreased urination. Babies should have at least a little wet diaper every six hours; older children should visit the bathroom at least every eight hours. The most important symptom of dehydration is listlessness and less interest in drinking. This is when you must call your pediatrician, or head directly to the emergency room.

Call If Your Child Is Acting Really Ill

Really ill can mean listless, disinterested, or not responding to you; it also means any child who can't be awakened easily. It includes children whose color is bad—pale, grey, or blue. Really ill children act very differently from their usual behavior. Please call us.

Call If Your Child Is in Unbearable Pain

Treat your child's pain—be it from an earache, skinned elbow, or anything else—with acetaminophen or ibuprofen routinely. They both work well, though ibuprofen should not be used in babies less than six months old. You should also try local measures like a cool compress for a bruised knee, or some hot tea for an older child with a sore throat. If these simple home remedies and medicines help substantially, then the pain is not caused by anything serious enough to warrant an after-hours phone call. But if after trying these measures your child is still visibly in pain and unable to sleep, call your pediatrician for more advice.

Call If You're Really Worried

Parents have a sense of what's right and wrong with their child. If parents are really worried, they should feel comfortable calling their pediatrician at any time. If your pediatrician has given you the impression that these calls aren't worth his time, you ought to find your children a new doctor.

Call for Anything Involving a Newborn

Newborns are tricky. Even I don't trust them, and I don't expect their exhausted parents to wait until morning. Any call from any parent with a newborn is fair game. Did I already mention we chose this profession?

Don't Call for Any Administrative or Insurance Matter

I know your HMO requires a referral from your primary doctor for you to be seen in the emergency room. I also know that the employees of your HMO are tucked away snoring in their little beds, and I don't have their home phone numbers. You should double-check the policy of your own pediatric practices, but most of us don't want to be awakened for purely administrative or insurance matters. Call the office in the morning; we'll get it straightened out then.

Don't Call for Routine Refills

It's rude to call for refills of medicines that can wait until tomorrow; it's also dangerous, because we don't typically have any way of double-checking the dose and accuracy of your child's medicines. Call during regular business hours when charts are available for routine medication refills. There are only a handful of medicines that absolutely must be taken every day—heart pills, for instance—and if your child is on these medicines you should make absolutely certain you don't get all the way to the bottom of the bottle before calling.

Don't Call for Any Long-Term Problem That Is Stable

If your child has had the same headache every day for two weeks, there is no reason to call tonight to talk about it. Likewise, problems that are chronic that are already being evaluated shouldn't be the subject of late-night calls unless there's truly a new development. Your pediatrician won't have any new insights or laboratory results when they're not at the office. Call tomorrow.

HOW TO CALL

Call your pediatrician's regular office number. There may be a telephone tree—listen for something like "Press 7 to page the doctor on call." Press whatever it takes to get to a person. Keep in mind that the operator will not be a nurse or anyone else medically trained. Just give a brief description of the problem, along with your child's name and birthday, and whatever phone numbers are best to reach you for the next hour or so. If you have a cell number, give that in addition to your home number. And as soon as you hang up disable anonymous call rejection on your home phone if you have that feature. (In the United States, dial *87.)

> ☞ **One cause of delayed return phone calls is anonymous call rejection. You may not even realize you have that feature on your phone line, but it will prevent your doctor from calling you back.**

WHEN TO CALL AGAIN

You already called, the doctor was paged, yet you haven't been called back? First, check your phone to make sure it's accepting calls, and again be sure to turn off anonymous call rejection. If it's been longer than reasonable, say more than thirty minutes for most issues, call the office and have the doctor paged again. Pagers aren't perfect, telephones aren't perfect, and pediatricians aren't perfect. If I receive more than one call within the same minute or two, I'm likely to forget to go back and return the first one. Make sure to tell the operator that it's your second attempt.

Remember that if you're really worried, take your child to the nearest hospital emergency department even if you haven't heard from your doctor yet. You can call the office and give them a cell number if you'll be better reached in your car.

WHAT TO TELL THE DOCTOR

Keep in mind that the doctor returning the call probably doesn't have access to your child's medical records. Even if it's your regular pediatrician who is on call that evening, assume that whomever you're speaking with doesn't know your child very well. If there is a complex past medical history, be prepared to summarize. Don't be insulted if you have to jog your pediatrician's memory.

Focus on the symptoms that have made you worry. When did the cough start? Exactly how high is the fever? How many times has he thrown up? Try to avoid guessing a diagnosis—"He has strep throat, I just know it"—and concentrate on the symptoms that are occurring. That will best help you and your pediatrician get to the most important facts.

Know your child's medication allergies, and know what medications are already being taken. Again, medical records are not available at night, so knowing "he's already on some antibiotic" isn't as helpful as "he's on amoxicillin, two teaspoons twice a day, and he started this three days ago." You should also know your child's weight. Your pediatrician will need this information to choose the correct dose of any needed medication.

Before your doctor calls, you should already have a pharmacy number handy. If it's after about 9:00 PM, your usual pharmacy is probably closed. Every family should have the number of the closest twenty-four-hour pharmacy handy. On holidays, you should call the pharmacy to make sure they're open before you give the number to your doctor.

> ☞ **You'll get more out of phone calls if you're prepared. Tell a brief story, focus on the symptoms that worry you most, and have your child's weight, allergies, and pharmacy number ready.**

COMMON SYMPTOMS THAT TRIGGER CALLS

This section is meant to guide you through some of the most common reasons why I've been called after business hours, along with a simple approach to knowing which of these children need urgent evaluation. While these tips are not meant as comprehensive information about these problems, you'll get some idea of what to do until your pediatrician's office opens the following morning.

Abdominal Pain

The most concerning abdominal pain is severe and relentless, leaving the child doubled over and unwilling to move. One good way to tell if your child's stomachache needs a doctor's input quickly is to gently squeeze the abdomen. Don't ask if it hurts, just observe how your child reacts to a gentle poke or squeeze to the belly. If there's a wince or a noticeable increase of pain when you push, you ought to be speaking with your doctor right away. On the other hand, if your child can walk up stairs or jump without much pain, the bellyache can probably wait.

Asthma

This is a very common cause of breathing trouble, and leads to many phone calls. If your child has asthma and has a wheeze or more than a mild cough, try their "rescue medication" [usually albuterol or levalbuterol (Xopenex)]. If these medicines are only a few months past their expiration dates, use them anyway; if you've run out completely, call the doctor. If after a single treatment there is still audible wheezing or any trouble breathing, try a second treatment fifteen minutes later. If after that your child is still wheezing, call the doctor. If the treatment did ease the wheezing, continue treatments about every four hours until the next day when you can contact your doctor for more specific plans. Note that children with more severe asthma should probably have oral steroid medications at home for emergencies; discuss emergency plans for the use of steroids with your pediatrician at your next routine visit.

Bleeding

If something is bleeding, put pressure on it. If it's in the mouth and difficult to press, try giving your child a popsicle to enjoy. If it's still oozing fifteen to thirty minutes later, the wound may need to be closed. Depending on circumstances and location, a doctor can use stitches, staples, glue, or bandages to best close different kinds of wounds; call your pediatrician for guidance on the best place to go. Any wound that is wide will end up with a scar unless the edges can be held together, so consider a trip to the ER for closure of cosmetically important wounds if they're gaping at all. Wounds of the tongue, gums, and inside of the lips rarely need stitches unless they're really deep or if they cross onto the face. Call your pediatrician for more specific guidance if you're not sure whether a wound needs stitches.

Broken Bones

A bone that's visibly broken needs to be treated right away; a hurt extremity that might be broken can wait until the next day if the injury was mild and the pain can be managed at home. For swollen things that hurt after an injury, apply ice for fifteen minutes out of every hour. More details about the initial steps to take after a bone injury are in Chapter 2, under "Orthopedic Surgeons."

Cold Symptoms

Cold symptoms can annoy both children and parents, but rarely in themselves indicate any serious problems unless the child is having trouble breathing. Cold medicines are not terribly effective, but for children older than two years they might be worth a try. Simple remedies—cough drops, popsicles, a humidifier, hot tea, extra fluids—can help as much as any medicine for symptoms of the common cold. For babies less than a year, saline nose drops are the best way to unstuff little noses.

Cough

A coughing child can keep everyone awake. Humidity and popsicles can help, and don't forget to restart asthma medications if your child has had problems with this in the past. If a miserable cough is keeping your child up, you can try an over-the-counter suppressant. Benadryl tends to be the most sedating of these products, which is usually exactly what families are looking for!

Diarrhea

Diarrhea, if unaccompanied by vomiting, is rarely a cause of serious dehydration in the developed world where there is good access to clean drinks. Children with diarrhea should be encouraged to drink whatever they want, as much as they want. See below for more information about vomiting if your child has both of these problems.

Ear Pain

Ear pain is most often caused by either a middle ear infection ("otitis media", or simply "ear infection"), or swimmer's ear ("otitis externa"). More rarely ear pain can occur with tooth problems, foreign things in the ear canal, or for no reason at all. It's impossible to know exactly what the cause is over the phone. To help an ear feel better, use a heating pad and a dose of acetaminophen or ibuprofen. If you have numbing drops, you can also use these—but not if there is visible ear drainage. Also, avoid putting in ear drops if you're going to see the doctor within the next few hours. Drops make it hard for us to see! If you do see pus in the ear canal, your child may have had a burst eardrum. Relax, that's not an emergency, they heal fine. Go see your pediatrician the next day.

Fever

Based on my informal review of all of the phone calls I received in my last weekend on call, fever was the most common complaint. Keeping things simple and brief, there are really only a few things you need to know about fevers in the middle of the night.

As reviewed in more detail in Chapter 5, fevers should be measured correctly or it's difficult to judge what to do about them. For babies less than three months, most of us prefer a rectal temperature be performed because that's the "standard." That is, pediatricians know how to interpret the exact number, and studies done on young babies with fever are always based on rectal temperatures. Once babies are older, an axillary (armpit) temperature is fine. Most five year olds can keep an oral thermometer under their tongues. Ear thermometers are unreliable at every age and should not be used. One new method that has promise is the "temporal artery" thermometer that quickly measures temperature with a pass over the forehead. Though I don't trust them yet for the littlest babies, they seem to be fine for three months and up.

Communicate clearly what the fever is. Don't add a degree and don't subtract a degree. Just report the thermometer's reading, and how you took it. If you didn't actually measure the temperature, be honest. It's fair to say "I didn't measure his temperature, but he feels really hot." If it's necessary to know the number, your doctor will ask you to measure it.

Fever itself will not harm your child. I know it's commonly thought that there's some magic number: a fever beyond which brain damage or death will occur. That's just not true. In the past, before vaccinations and antibiotics, high fevers would often herald a deadly illness—that's what grandma remembers, and that's why prior generations are so frightened of fever. But it was never the fever itself that did the harm; it was the underlying cause of the fever. And thanks to vaccines, these have changed to far less terrifying problems.

(To be complete: in dehydrated athletes with "heat stroke," high fevers can cause brain damage or death. Their temperatures can exceed 107°F, and they are very ill. This occurs only when overheating, overexertion, and dehydration occur together. It is not what wakes your child up with fever at night.)

Though fever itself doesn't hurt children, it will make them feel lousy: headachy, grumpy, and listless. During a fever, a child's breathing and pulse will also be fast. When your child has a fever, treat her with either ibuprofen or acetaminophen at the correct dose. You can also use a tepid water bath—never cold water, and absolutely never rubbing alcohol. Once the fever comes down, you'll be able to more accurately gauge how sick your child really is.

> ☞ **How sick is your child? You'll get a more accurate picture *after* giving fever medicine.**

Beyond the important issue of helping your child feel better, fevers themselves are caused by something. The question in the middle of the night is: does my child need to be evaluated for this right now? In other words, what is the chance that the fever is caused by a serious problem that can't wait until morning?

There are several key factors that can help you and your pediatrician decide the likelihood or a serious problem causing the fever:

- *Age.* The younger a child, the more likely fever is something serious. A baby less than two or three months with a fever over 100.8°F rectally needs to be evaluated right away. Older infants and certainly children can usually wait until morning, unless there is more to the story.
- *How they act when the fever is down.* This is crucial. When children have a fever of 103°F, they look and act sick. Unless you can't wait to head to the ER, give the child a dose of fever medicine, and wait thirty minutes. If the fever goes down and the child perks up and acts much better than it is very unlikely that there is a serious infection. Evaluation can wait until the next day. But if after fever medicine the child still looks really lousy, head to the ER. Sometimes I'll tell a family to give a dose of ibuprofen on the way to the ER, so if in the waiting room the medicine kicks in and the child perks up, the family can go back home and see me in the morning.
- *Risk factors.* Children with serious immune problems (for example chemotherapy, sickle cell anemia, or immunodeficiency syndromes) are far more worrisome when they run fevers. If your child has a condition like one of these,

you should already have a specific fever action plan in place so you know exactly what to do.

- *Vaccinations.* Once your child has received two doses of vaccines (that is, by four months), there's good protection against bloodstream infections and meningitis, two of the most serious causes of fevers. If for any reason your child has not received these vaccines, there is a higher likelihood that fevers are associated with life-threatening infections. Tell the pediatrician who calls you back if your child has missed routine vaccinations.

Pink Eye

The things to watch out for are a lot of swelling around the eye, or a strong feeling that there's something in the eye itself. If these things are going on, the child needs to be evaluated. But for the more ordinary case where the white of the eye is pink and there's some goo, it's usually either infectious ("pink eye") or allergic. Kids who have gooey but white eyes do not have pink eye; in other words, pink eye has got to be pink! Some pediatricians will be happy to call in eye drops if the diagnosis is straightforward. Although day-care centers act as if pink eye is deadly serious, ordinary pink eye really isn't a big deal. It causes much less misery than a common cold, which is just as contagious.

Rashes

Rashes are tough to diagnose over the phone, but a few quick insider tips can help:

- If it itches and it's small, try topical hydrocortisone ointment.
- If it itches and it's big, try oral Benadryl.
- See if the rash blanches. That is, press your thumbs on either side of a rash, and stretch the skin. If the rash goes away with stretching then comes back when you release your thumbs, the rash is "blanching." In general, rashes that blanch are very unlikely to be anything serious enough to warrant an ER visit.
- If the rash doesn't blanch, call your doctor right away.
- The rules at the beginning of the chapter apply to rashes, too. That is, a rash in a child that's acting ill needs attention no matter what else is going on.

Vomiting

It isn't the vomiting, per se, that ends up causing trouble; it's dehydration. As we've said, your child is much more likely to get dehydrated if vomiting is accompanied by diarrhea and/or fever. Review the earlier section about dehydration so you know what to look for.

Parents are sometimes surprised to learn that there are no good medicines approved for use in treating nausea in young children. Phenergan has been used, though there's a risk of breathing problems and sedation and it is specifically contraindicated for use in children less than two. The newest medicine to try is Zofran, which is designed for children with nausea from chemotherapy. It seems to be very safe and effective for vomiting down to age one, but it is very expensive and not FDA-approved for this use.

A slow-and-steady approach is better than medicine when your child is vomiting. Continuously offer little tiny sips of fluids. Ideally, use a balanced electrolyte solution such as Pedialyte; for older kids a sports drink like Gatorade is a reasonable and better-tasting alternative. Avoid using red liquids that could fool you into thinking that vomit or diarrhea has blood in it. The key is to offer little sips at a time, just one teaspoon every ten minutes for little babies and one ounce at a time for teens. Even if there's persistent vomiting, as long as your child continues to take these little sips dehydration can be prevented. Head to the ER if sips are refused and there are signs of dehydration. And wash your hands—the only thing worse than a vomiting child is when parents start vomiting, too.

> **The best treatment for vomiting is frequent, small sips of appropriate fluids. This is more important and more effective in preventing complications than any medicine.**

Kids get sick at odd times, and telephone calls are inevitable. You should be able to trust your pediatrician to give you good advice that doesn't always include a trip to the ER. If you think you've really got an emergency on your hands, give your pediatrician a call for guidance. Parents and pediatricians both sleep better when they know the kids are OK.

This chapter is meant to provide general guidelines for when and how to contact your pediatrician for after-hours care. You cannot rely on this or any other published material to provide exact advice for every situation. If you are ever worried that your child is ill, contact your physician.

7

AN INSIDE LOOK AT EMERGENCY ROOMS AND HOSPITALS

The emergency room (ER) can be the most exciting place to work as a health care provider, and the most miserable place to be as a parent. An ER will accept everyone, from children with life-threatening emergencies to children in nearly perfect health. On a busy night there might be a homeless runaway alongside a newborn whose insurance-mandated early discharge prevented detection of a heart defect. With luck, you'll never have to take your child to the ER. But parents should be prepared not only for an ER visit, but also for the possibility that their child will someday have to be admitted to the hospital.

This chapter takes an insider's look at ER and hospital care for children. You'll learn what you need to know to be ready for an ER visit and how to get good care throughout any hospital encounter.

BE PREPARED

Ask your pediatrician in advance where you ought to take you child for emergency care. In some communities, pediatric-only hospitals have their own ERs to handle sick kids; in other places children are seen at general community hospitals that may have a set-off area of their main ER for children. Your pediatrician will know what facility is best at handling the needs of young patients.

Your city may have "urgent care centers" or "immediate care centers" in addition to conventional ERs at hospitals. These free-standing facilities are often derisively called "doc-in-the-boxes." They are designed to handle after-hours care of

> ☞ **Find out from your pediatrician, now, where the best pediatric after-hours facilities are. Believe me, your pediatrician will know which places do good medicine and which places are to be avoided.**

routine problems, but are not truly emergency departments. They're not open twenty-four hours, and don't have the facilities to handle genuine emergency medical problems. Many are ill-equipped to see children. Ask your pediatrician if your local "doc-in-the-box" offers good care that you can rely on after hours.

If your child seems ill enough to warrant an emergency visit, you'll probably want to call your pediatrician first to confirm that you really need to go and to find out the best facility that's available for your problem. Your pediatrician might be able to call in to the ER to give them background information, especially if your child has a complex medical history. Note, however, that your pediatrician will *not* be able to get you seen faster by making a phone call. ERs work by seeing the sickest kids first, and there's no way of knowing how many children with more serious problems may need to be seen ahead of you.

Bring toys, books, movies, a portable DVD player—anything to pass the time. Bring any medications your child is taking, and all of your insurance information. Any sibling should be left at home if possible, ideally with a sitter so both parents can be available to accompany the sick child. It will be a long, boring trip, and you'll want two adults to help keep your child as comfortable as possible. Two adults are also better able to keep on top of questions and instructions from the ER doctors.

Food and Drink in the ER

Kids can sure get cranky when they're hungry! But not every child in the ER should be having snacks. Follow these rules to avoid causing problems or a delay with your child's care:

- Vomiting children should only be offered small sips of liquids. For babies, a balanced electrolyte solution like Pedialyte is best, but older kids can sip Gatorade or a similar sports drink.
- Children with severe belly pain should be given nothing to eat or drink until they've been evaluated.
- Children who may need to be sedated (for sutures or for a CT scan) should be given nothing to eat or drink.
- Children who may need surgery should also be given nothing to eat or drink. This might include a child with a badly broken bone, a child with appendicitis, or a child with an incarcerated (stuck) hernia.

It can be hard to know if it's a good idea to offer your children snacks or drinks in the ER, so it's usually best to ask when you get there.

AT THE ER

The most frustrating part of any ER encounter is the wait. But keep in mind that if you have a long wait, it's because *other children are sicker than yours.* If you hear a story about a child who upon arrival at the ER was immediately pounced on by three nurses and two doctors, that's not a good thing—that child was very, very ill.

When you meet the physician who'll be seeing your child, be sure to get a name, ideally printed on a card with contact information. While talking with the doctors and nurses, be honest, thorough, and focused on exactly what symptoms made you bring your child to the ER.

You may wonder what to do during a potentially painful procedure such as suturing or starting an intravenous line. I think it's best if parents stay in the room to console the child, but some doctors may not be comfortable with this depending on the nature of the procedure. Talk directly with the doctor about the best place for you to be to help your child relax without interfering with the physician's work. All parents should sit down during medical procedures—I once had a mom faint while I sutured up her son's chin. (Actually, the child thought it was kind of funny. So did I . . . afterwards!)

> ☞ **As frustrating as it may be to wait, you don't want to be the parents of the child who is seen quickly in the ER.**

When it's time to leave, be sure to take copies of all laboratory reports, x-rays, and any other notes that are available. If your child was seen by multiple physicians or specialists, get all of their names and contact information. You should know the exact plan for follow-up with your own pediatrician and any specialists who may have become involved.

IF YOUR CHILD IS ADMITTED

Your child might need to stay at the hospital overnight, or longer. Some inside tips will help you keep your child comfortable, and will help you keep track of what's going on.

Try to keep your child comfortable. Bring favorite toys, stuffed animals, and movies. Unless your child has a gastrointestinal issue requiring a special diet, you should be able to bring in some favorite foods. Adults should accompany children while they're in the hospital at all times, but parents should try to take turns with spouses or other trusted adults to get some breaks. A well-rested adult can help console a child better, and will be better able to stay on top of medical information and decisions.

Know who is responsible for your child's care, and how to contact that person. The main doctor during a hospitalization is called an "attending physician," or simply "attending." If your own pediatrician follows inpatients, the attending may be someone you know well; but many practices rely on inpatient-dedicated physicians called "hospitalists" to take care of any children who are admitted from their practice. In teaching hospitals, your attending may be assisted by doctors-in-training called "residents" or "interns". Though they have medical degrees and will be called "Dr. So-and-so," they have not completed their training and are not the ones responsible for your child's care. Make sure that your most important questions and concerns are addressed by your child's attending physician. Likewise, if specialists are called in to assist they may have their own residents and assistants. Know names and contact information for both your main attending and any specialists so you can contact them during or after the hospitalization.

If your own pediatricians aren't directly involved in your child's inpatient care, call their office in the morning to let them know you're in the hospital. Some ERs admit children directly to the inpatient wards without calling the community pediatrician, so it's possible your usual doctors don't know what happened. They may want to visit the hospital just to keep in touch. If you have HMO-style insurance, your primary pediatrician may be required to contact your insurance carrier. In fact, because hospital bills can quickly become huge, contact your insurance carrier yourself on the first business day after hospitalization to confirm all steps have been taken to ensure coverage.

Many parents never have to take a child to an ER, and certainly never have to accompany them during a hospital admission. But if your child needs this level of care, you'll need to keep a clear head. With this chapter in mind you should be better prepared to help your child at the time when you're needed most.

8

HAPPY PATIENTS, HAPPY DOCTOR

Doctors want happy patients. Believe me, my staff and nurses have no desire to make you upset, and it is far easier to communicate with a happy child than a screaming one. Sometimes, though, things happen to disappoint families and upset the children. In this chapter we'll go through a list of the top common complaints from a pediatric office, and what you can do about them.

Most of these frustrating problems are best addressed at the visit by the patient or parents speaking up and voicing their concerns. You should feel comfortable asking your doctor about these issues—if you don't, you need another doctor. If you've tried to address these concerns and you aren't seeing any improvement, move on to a new pediatrician.

You've got a problem with something that occurred at the pediatrician's office. Who should you talk to?

- Nurse or receptionist? For a minor issue, it's always better to talk immediately with whoever is involved. But if you've got a serious gripe, you need to go to the boss.
- The business or office manager? This individual oversees the staff in most offices, and is a good person to talk with about a staff or nurse problem. The business manager has little sway on the doctors themselves.
- Your own favorite pediatrician? This is the single best individual to talk with about things that are disappointing you about the office. Your own pediatrician has the most interest in keeping you happy. If your family has been a patient for years, your pediatrician will be very willing to take your criticism seriously and try to help you out.
- The physician-owner? Most practices are owned by one or more of the senior pediatricians. These owners certainly have an interest in keeping the customers happy, but traditionally doctors don't criticize

other doctors in the group unless there has been a big screw-up. If you just love the practice but feel that your doctor has let you down in some way, you can try to contact the owner-physician for redress. This might be especially useful if you're criticizing a doctor new to the group. Of course, your own pediatrician and the owner may turn out to be one and the same person!

SOME TOP COMPLAINTS

The Doctor Didn't Listen

Minds wander, and this may well be true. Try to help the doctor listen by sticking to your main problem. You and the pediatrician need to keep focused, which may be especially difficult with an active child exploring the room. If the doctor does not seem to be paying attention, try to get the visit back on track by stating something like "I'm not sure we're following each other. My main concern is. . . ."

The Doctor Didn't Fix the Problem

Perhaps the doctor has a different perception of what the problem is. At a recheck appointment, the ear infection may look better through an otoscope. But if the baby still isn't sleeping, from the parent's point of view the problem may not be solved. Some problems are complex, and it may take more than one visit to adjust medications or otherwise reach a solution. Be realistic in what you expect doctors to accomplish. If you're frustrated by the pace of evaluation and treatment, speak up so you can understand what sort of recovery is expected.

My Child Got Upset

Doctor's offices can be a scary place, especially when you are a child who doesn't feel well. If you have a child who finds the pediatrician's office upsetting, try to defuse the situation when your child isn't already sick and upset. Stop by the office for a quick hello and wave, and get your own play doctor equipment so Junior can practice on a stuffed animal. Some children can certainly be more challenging than others. Your pediatrician should be willing to spend some extra time helping an anxious child settle down. Feel free to suggest any of these, and keep in mind that most pediatricians have plenty of their own tricks, too!

- Try the exam in a parent's lap. I routinely do this for children from six months to four years or so. The mental association I want them to keep is that as long as they're in a parent's lap, no harm will come to them. The table is the place for the ouchies—but at least it's only a brief time up there, and once they can get down the child can feel safe again.

- Try the exam in an office or waiting room rather than in an exam room.
- Try to do the entire encounter outside. I've got some nice steps beside my office door, and some kids are so tickled to see the doctor outside they forget to be upset.
- Let mom or dad, or even the child herself, help with the exam. I'll let mom hold the stethoscope to the chest, or let dad help manipulate an injured knee while I watch. Kids can hold the otoscope themselves to look in my ears first; then they often won't mind holding it in their own ears so I can take a peek. Most kids are more than happy to point a flashlight into their own mouths.

If none of this works, there is a time for just holding the child tightly while the exam gets done. I try to move quickly and efficiently through this, and use the tough-love approach only as a last resort. You can get a good look in an ear through sheer force, but it doesn't make the next visit go any better!

The Doctor Didn't Prescribe What Was Wanted

This may be because of unreasonable expectations (for example, you want an antibiotic for a viral infection), or it might be because the doctor didn't know you wanted specific item. You should tell the doctor if you didn't get what you expected. You may still leave without it, but you should get an explanation.

The "Wrong" Diagnosis Was Suggested

Sometimes parents come in already having decided what the diagnosis ought to be, and are disappointed that the doctor didn't agree. Perhaps the parents recall that a similar illness was diagnosed differently in the past, or their neighbor's child with the same symptoms was given a different diagnosis by their doctor. Maybe a parent has already been diagnosed with one thing, and their child with similar symptoms is thought by the pediatrician to have something else. In cases like this, speak up! The physician certainly doesn't want you to leave angry, and would welcome an opportunity to explain how a diagnosis is reached.

Sometimes, the diagnosis that best fits a child's symptoms is psychiatric or behavioral in nature. A good doctor will appreciate that many physical symptoms have a psychologic cause, and will be willing to bring this up. For instance, a teenager with chronic headaches may well have a main diagnosis of depression, rather than a more "medical" diagnosis. Keep in mind that the headaches are real and debilitating, and it doesn't do anyone any good to avoid dealing with a serious problem like depression while running from doctor to doctor for more and more tests. Most doctors are very reluctant to suggest a psychiatric or behavioral disorder, partially because they do not want to offend parents. If your physician is brave enough to bring this up as a possibility, you ought to take it seriously.

The Doctor Was Rude

It happens! Why? Here are some possibilities:

- The doctor is a jerk. Let's face it, medical school is designed for people who can rise to the top of a class, read for hours on end, and stay upright without sleep. In other words, a medical student isn't necessarily a nice person. I like to think that pediatrics attracts the more friendly, happier types of medical students, but a few rotten ones are bound to slip by.
- The doctor is tired, or having a bad day, or both. I usually don't tell, but there is a possibility I didn't sleep at all last night, and I might be preoccupied because of a bad diagnosis I have to discuss with some parents over lunch. There is often far more going on in the doctor's head than what's in the exam room.
- The doctor feels pressed for time. It may not be your fault, or your doctor's fault, but a waiting room full of customers upset about the wait can make your doctor and the staff anxious, too. Focus and forge ahead.
- Your child might be acting like a demon. Dealing with a child who's scared and screaming is expected to happen occasionally, especially at the toddler age, but if your child is still pitching a fit at age three it will wear a bit thin. And from any age child, getting kicked in the crotch will put a doctor in a sour mood. It might be that this particular doctor's style is not bringing out the best in your child. If it happens every time, it might be time to change doctors.

In any case, if you feel that the doctor is being rude, ask yourself if it's just an isolated incident. If it happens often, find another physician.

The Staff or a Nurse Was Rude

Again, sometimes it's just someone having a bad day, or sometimes you run across someone who just isn't suited to dealing with people. If it is an isolated, minor incident, you might let it pass. But if an employee of mine is making you uncomfortable, I certainly want to know. Please tell the doctor or business manager if an employee is rude or in any other way unprofessional.

The Doctor Took the Wrong Side in an Argument

I personally try to be very sensitive about these situations—I am not a marriage counselor. Especially for problems like sleep training, potty training, and feeding issues, I'll try to ask both parents what they think they should do before I say anything; this avoids a lot of hurt feelings. Sometimes, the pediatrician has to make the call, and sometimes a parent feels shorted. Sorry about that.

The Wait Was Too Long

I hate waiting for doctors, too, and I know that a long wait before even seeing the doctor can ruin the encounter before it begins. Avoid the wait by choosing appointment times first thing in the morning or first thing after lunch; always avoid the last few appointments of the day if possible. Bring toys and books. You can also bring reasonable snacks that distract the little ones, like drinks from sippy cups or crackers and cookies in little baggies so they don't end up all over the place. (But don't go overboard. I've walked into exam rooms where a family literally has a picnic lunch spread out on the floor! It is not reasonable to expect nurses to clean up after your kids' meals, and eating in medical care areas is forbidden under federal occupational safety rules.) Understand that some waits are going to occur in the best run practices. If the wait is always too long, switch to another doctor. In the next chapter, we'll reveal the inside secrets about why there's such a wait at many doctors' offices, along with more tips on how to schedule your visits to avoid a long wait.

9

SCHEDULING TO YOUR ADVANTAGE AND OTHER OFFICE TRICKS

Parents and their kids hate waiting for the doctor. The waiting room is boring and filled with sick children; once you get back to an exam room, it can get even worse. Why are doctors always late? And is there anything families can do to avoid the wait?

Of course, dealing with your child's health care entails more than just visits to your doctor. The staff and nurses will often be your main contact point for getting things you need quickly. With an insider's help, you can learn how to avoid both the hassle of waiting and other useful tips on getting what you need from your pediatrician's office.

WHY THE WAIT?

There are several reasons, some of which might surprise you.

The Insurance Company Wants You to Wait

Insurance companies pay for most doctor visits. From their point of view, each visit costs them more. They do not want you going to the doctor unnecessarily, so it is in their interests to make going to the doctor at least a little bit inconvenient and difficult. If seeing a doctor was as easy as dropping by a convenience store, the insurance company would have to spend far more money on your health care. What exactly constitutes an "unnecessary" visit is debatable, of course. But as far as the payer goes, it's usually better to discourage visits and hope things work out for the best.

How does the insurance company encourage doctors to make patients wait? They pay a relatively small amount for each visit, or in some cases do not pay at all. A pediatrician has to see a large number of patients a day to cover overhead and try to turn a profit. To get many patients seen, the schedule is designed to be "tight." That means there's little time allotted for each patient, and typically zero time allotted between patients for catching up and for emergencies. Doctors often overbook, with more than one patient scheduled for each time block. This helps keep the physician busy even if someone is late or misses an appointment. Scheduling tricks like these are designed to get the maximum number of patients seen, which works to the physician's advantage. They are not designed to minimize your wait.

Doctors Have Emergencies

This is true, even if the excuse might be overused in some offices. Sometimes kids are brought in genuinely ill, with difficulty breathing or a seizure. The physician and the staff must instantly respond to the emergency, to the detriment of patients waiting. I've been asked: why not schedule time for emergencies? Because you never know when they'll occur!

Doctors Have Other "Unschedulable Responsibilities"

Answering phone calls and reviewing and signing last minute "I have to get this done NOW or Johnny can't go to camp" forms all take up time when the doctor should be in the exam rooms. But again, this time is difficult to schedule into the day. And doctors do not want to set aside time for activities that do not generate revenue.

Patients Do Not Always Take a Predictable Amount of Time

This is the number one reason why I sometimes can't stay on schedule. My main job is to evaluate and begin to treat every concern parents bring to me, in addition to keeping an eye out for unsuspected problems and counseling to prevent future problems. Keeping all of this in mind for every patient means that there is just no way to know how long a visit will take.

Phil and Jill: A Tale of Two Coughs

Two back to back appointments were made for ten-year-olds who came mostly for cough. But it turns out that these "simple" visits took vastly different turns, and one took up far more time than the other.

Phil had an upper respiratory infection with a cough that was keeping him awake. We talked for ten minutes, mostly about ways to keep him comfortable at night.

Jill also came in to see me for cough. It turns out her cough was mostly occurring on weekends when she visited her daddy. He didn't "believe" in her asthma medications; he also had a live-in girlfriend who smoked. It turns out that his having this girlfriend at his apartment was news to the mom, and it violated the court order about parental visitation. Mom was reluctant to further criticize dad in front of the child, but she motioned me outside on the pretense of needing to review the bill. While in my office she privately wondered about other inappropriate behavior that was going on at her ex-husband's place. After thirty minutes, we still hadn't really solved the problem of Jill's cough, and I had to ask mom to return at another time so I could talk to Jill more about life at dad's on weekends. I also left a note to myself to call dad over lunch to hear his side of the story—though I'll probably work through lunch to make up the time spent on this visit!

Jill's case is not unique; visits for "simple" complaints can turn into the longest encounters of my day. But a good pediatrician will help parents feel that they can talk about things that take extra time. Don't be too upset if occasionally you have to wait with your simple Phil at the doctor's office. Some other time, you're going to bring in a complex Jill, and you'll be glad that your pediatrician takes the extra time with you when you need it.

A good office will try to schedule extra time for a known complex patient or problem, but there is often no way to know before walking into an exam room how much time evaluation and management will take. I tell my patients that I will try to spend as much time as necessary with everyone, which means that if you are next in line after a suicidal teenager with two years of headaches and a rash and divorcing parents, you are in for a long wait. And what do you think happens to my schedule if two time-intensive patients happen to come in a row?

Some offices try to overcome this problem by using a designated "scheduler" rather than allowing any receptionist to make appointments. The scheduler may be a nurse, or a highly trained receptionist. The advantage is that this person spends time with each caller to help more exactly identify the amount of time that might be needed, which might help keep the physician on schedule better. However, there is a huge disadvantage to this system: during busy times, you'll usually have to leave a message for the scheduler to call you back, and you may end up with a prolonged game of phone tag to get your appointment. This system is more common in adult groups than in pediatrics, because kids have so many immediate-need, same-day appointments that using a single person as a scheduler is not practical.

Some Patients Come in at the Wrong Time, or with No Appointment at All

Walk-ins and late patients can wreak havoc on the most carefully planned schedule. Sometimes these patients still have to be seen, especially if the child is genuinely sick or the parents are especially worried. A well-run office will look for patterns, and if one family is always late or always misses appointments, they will be asked to leave the practice.

HOW TO AVOID THE WAIT

- Look for a well-run practice with conscientious doctors who try to stay on time. If you *always* wait ninety minutes to see the doctor, they are not trying hard enough to stay in control of the schedule. Of course, if you *never* have to wait, it means that the doctor either has barely any business or does not prolong the visits of complex patients. In other words, a practice where you *never* have to wait may not be ideal, either.
- When the schedule is running behind, a good practice will try several things to keep families happy. Look for a practice that is willing to move appointments, or offer for waiting patients to try to see another doctor. At the least, you should be kept informed of what's going on.
- Try to get one of the first appointments of the day, or one of the first appointments after lunch. The timing of later appointments is more likely to be thrown off by the accumulated issues that come up throughout the day.
- Be on time, or even a few minutes early, especially for an early appointment.
- Avoid going to the doctor on the busiest days: Monday is the worst, followed by Friday. Also, on single day school holiday like a teacher's workday, no one bothers to travel. You might think it would be a good day to get a check up done, but it is not. Everyone else has already thought of this, and these days are notoriously hectic.
- If you have a complex problem, especially one that involves a lengthy explanation of a social or school situation, mention it to a scheduler. If you have a medical problem that you think might take a lot of time, ask to discuss this with a nurse prior to the visit.
- Do not try to lump in a sibling's issues with a scheduled visit. If you've scheduled a visit for one child, expect the doctor to help you with her issues. It is not reasonable to expect the doctor to also spend time discussing or examining your other child. It is also not fair to your other child to get less than the doctor's full attention.
- In many practices some doctors tend to run more on time than others—maybe they're less busy, or maybe they have fewer appointment slots, or maybe they're less tolerant of phone interruptions and focus only on moving from room to room. If you know you need to get through the office in a hurry, book with the physician who most often runs on time. If you're new to the practice, you can discreetly ask the scheduler about which doctors tend to run on time. The scheduler will deny that anyone is really bad, but might nonetheless suggest who you should see.

If you always have an unreasonable wait, mention it to your physicians. They'll be more motivated to look at their schedule and at what they're doing if they hear it from the patients, especially if they hear it from familiar patients who aren't usually complainers. If the problem is persistently annoying, consider whether your attachment to that physician is worth the extra time.

OTHER TRICKS TO GET THE MOST OUT
OF YOUR DOCTOR'S OFFICE

Besides trying to avoid a wait, there are many other things that parents need to get done at their pediatrician's office. With an insider's help you'll find it easier get many other practical tasks accomplished.

I Need to Speak with My Doctor on the Phone

From my point of view, this is a tough one. Many, many parents want to speak with me directly to clarify advice or to give me follow-up on a problem, and I just do not have the time to take all of these calls personally. It's in part a financial decision: physicians do not traditionally charge for phone conversations, and any time I spend on the phone is time I could spend in an exam room, with a paying customer. If I were to return all of the calls that come in to me, I would not be able to stay in business.

But some phone calls really are best handled directly by the physician. Sometimes they're social or family problems, or problems that can't be discussed openly in front of a child. Sometimes it really does make more sense to speak with the doctor directly.

So what's the best way to get your doctor on the phone? Speak first with one of the nurses, and give a brief version of what's on your mind. Tell the nurse you feel you need to speak to your doctor directly. Give your phone numbers, including cell number, and several likely times you can be reached. And be flexible—remember that physicians get a lot of these calls, and you might have to wait a few days. If you haven't heard back in a reasonable time, call again. Be polite, but be sure to explain that you've needed to call more than once. If this still doesn't work, make an appointment to see the doctor, and slip a note to him or her directly. If you still can't get good communication, it may be time to change doctors.

I'd Like to Get Some Free Samples

Just ask. Doctor's offices get plenty of samples of name brand medicines, formula, and other health items. Feel free to ask a nurse or physician if there are samples available, especially if you've been prescribed a newer medication. Usually there are no samples of generic medicines.

I'm Having Trouble Paying My Bills

Please speak up if family or job troubles are making it difficult to make ends meet. If you keep in contact with the practice's business manager, I do not think any physician would ever refuse care or kick you out if you're having financial trouble. The key is to communicate and make some sincere effort to show you'd like to pay.

Also, let the physician know if money is a problem. We may be able to be more careful about ordering expensive medicines, or we may be able to load you up with samples.

I Need to Get This Form Signed Right Away

Please don't threaten to raise a stink if the physician isn't pulled out of a room immediately to sign your form. That won't work, and might get you dismissed from the practice. Be nice, be polite, explain, and be flexible. We don't want Johnny to miss camp either, and we'll get the form signed. If you're really in trouble and need something at the very last minute, bring a box of fresh donuts and a smile.

I Want to Have a Medication Called in without Being Seen

This can depend on the office; some have fairly liberal call-in policies, some consider it absolutely forbidden. Ask about that when you're deciding upon a practice. But a few general suggestions might help:

- *Know who to talk to.* If it's a clinical problem, you probably need to discuss it with a nurse, not a receptionist.
- *Be reasonable.* There are some times when you just need to come in to be evaluated.
- *Be honest.* It doesn't work to exaggerate the symptoms or severity—rather than encourage me to call in a prescription over the phone, I'm more likely to insist you come in. Just be honest and tell us exactly what is going on.
- *Have your pharmacy number handy.* I've had midnight phone calls where mom insists not only that I call in a medicine, but wants me to look up a pharmacy that's close to her and open at night.
- *Avoid the phrase "I know Dr. so-and-so would call it in!"* I know my partners, too, and I may well have your chart in front of me. Pitting the doctors of a group against each other might work once, but in the long run it will get you kicked out.
- *Be friendly.* As they say, you're more likely to catch flies with honey than with vinegar.

The key to many of these is to speak up honestly, concisely, and politely. A good pediatric office should be able to accommodate all of the above requests, at least most of the time. You should look for a group that helps you avoid most of the unnecessary waiting and is responsive to parents' requests.

10

MEDICINES: HOW TO CHOOSE THEM, HOW TO USE THEM

Doctors can choose from a huge array of medicines and other treatments. How do we decide which is best for your child? And once you've got a prescription, what's the best way to use these potent chemicals to get the most benefit with the least side effects?

Medical doctors and a few other professionals are empowered to prescribe medications. (Depending on state law, other well-trained professionals can prescribe as well, including dentists, nurse practitioners, some optometrists, and podiatrists.) It's thought that our extensive training and experience gives us the ability to judge who will best benefit from a prescription, and in what cases the risks of taking prescription drugs are justified. Though it may seem like an overwhelming subject, I encourage parents to try to understand the science behind medical studies and decisions. Even if you'd rather just let the doctor make the decisions, parents still need to know how to use these medicines in the best way.

How Doctors (Should) Choose Medicines

Doctors rely on personal experience, training, and routine to choose medications. There are also more sinister influences, like advertising and pleas from the drug sales force. But the most important, best reason to choose one drug over another is the science. What's really been proven to work best?

A multibillion dollar industry is behind the development and marketing of medicines. Funding for research and development comes not only from the drug companies, but also from the federal government, private charity groups, and academic institutions. New therapies undergo intense, thorough, and expensive studies long before they are approved and marketed. Despite this, there are some humbling truths that insiders know about medicine. You may be surprised to learn that the majority of healing for most ordinary pediatric illnesses has nothing to do with drugs, and that many medicines are only a little more effective than sugar pills.

Why is it important for you to understand how research is used to find out if a drug really works? Unfortunately, you cannot assume that your physician has the time or temperament to read new medical studies carefully. By understanding how to tell a good study from a bad study, you'll be able to tell if physicians know what they're talking about, or whether they're just reading the headlines. You'll also be better equipped to evaluate newspaper accounts of the newest medical research. Neither newspaper journalists nor editors of medical journals guarantee that any published account is valid, or applies to your family. Finally, many of my patients' families are reading the medical literature directly, and it is not difficult to understand the concepts that allow doctors or laymen to understand exactly what a study is really saying.

☞ **All new medicines carry more potential risk than older medicines because they don't have a track record proving their safety. Often, side effects and risks become apparent only after years of experience. To even consider taking a new drug, there should be adequate proof that it is more effective than older medicines.**

THE PROOF: DOES A MEDICINE WORK?

The best way to determine if a medication is going to be effective is through a clinical trial. Though there are variations depending on the nature of the medicine being studied, there are five essential steps of almost any good clinical trial:

1. *Selection:* Collect a group of children who all have the disease you are studying.
2. *Randomization:* Divide the group into two smaller groups, which should be as identical as possible.
3. *Treatment:* Give one group the new drug (often called the study drug). The children of the other group either get no drug at all or a dummy medicine (placebo).
4. *Blinding:* Neither the children, their families, nor the treating doctors and nurses should know who got the study drug and who got the placebo.
5. *Results:* Using some sort of objective measure, figure out whether the kids on the study drug did better than the kids on placebo in a significant way.

Every one of these steps is crucial, and every step is loaded with pitfalls that can make a study worthless. One reason that you've seen contradictory results about medical treatments in the newspaper is that it is difficult to perform a perfect clinical trial. Most published studies are far short of perfect, but insiders know that each of these five steps should be done well to convince a pediatrician that a new therapy is effective.

Step 1: Selection

For a study to be useful to me, the children involved in a study should be like the children in my practice. It may be interesting to see how children in

Bangladesh respond to a new therapy for diarrhea, but I know that my own patients may be very different in nutritional status, ethnic background, and overall health than Bangladeshi kids. Likewise, the age of the study participants is important. I can't assume that a therapy effective in teenagers will necessarily work on infants.

Not only should the children in a study be very much like my own patients, but the disease being studied should be exactly the disease I am trying to treat. A medicine that helps people with sore throat caused by *Streptococcus* bacteria may not help a person with a viral sore throat.

> ☞ **For a study to determine if a medicine is likely to help your child with a certain problem, the study participants must be similar to your child and must have the same problem.**

Step 2: Randomization

When the group of study participants is divided into two groups, one for the real medicine and one for the sham medicine, it is crucial that this be done randomly. If there is any hint that the people running the study, either intentionally or unintentionally, skewed the results by putting those with more severe disease disproportionally into one group, than the results are not valid.

To prove that the two groups were well randomized, a good study will include a table of the characteristics of the two groups, including age, sex, severity of disease, race, and other factors. As near as possible, all of these characteristics should be identical in the two groups in order to ensure an unbiased result that reflects a true difference between the study drug and placebo.

Step 3: Treatment

One group gets the study drug, and the other group gets "something else" for comparison. This "something else" might be an established treatment, a sugar pill (placebo), or no treatment at all. It's important that the study designers keep an eye on compliance. That is, all or at least close to all of the participants should take all of their medicine, as directed. If the study drug causes notable side effects, it may be more likely that kids in the study group will stop taking their medicine, which will tend to decrease any potential effectiveness. Also, the treatment should be exactly the medicine that is in question, and the exact same thing at the same dose your own doctor could prescribe.

Step 4: Blinding

As best as possible, neither the participants nor the people administering the study should know whether any individual patient is getting genuine experimental drug or placebo. If this is done correctly, the study is said to be "double blinded." The opposite of a blinded trial is an "open" trial, which may be useful for getting preliminary information but can never be a reliable indicator of effectiveness. Though double blinding isn't always practical, it is the best way to guard against bias. If either the patients or the doctors subconsciously change the way they perceive symptoms depending on whether they think they're getting medicine, the results will be biased and invalid. As we'll see later, a patient who *thinks* a real medicine is being given is much more likely to report that it worked, even if the medicine is really a placebo. Blinding is crucial in separating the real effect of medicine from "wishful thinking" among the patients and doctors involved in a study.

> ☞ Do not believe any *open* study that shows a new medicine is effective. New medicines are by their nature potentially more risky than established medicines, and only a blinded study provides the proof of effectiveness that justifies their additional risk.

Step 5: Results

The results of a study have to be measured objectively. How much did the blood pressure decrease? How quickly did the fever disappear? If the nature of the most important symptom is subjective, than some sort of independent scoring system has to be employed. Using this objective measure, the results of the study group versus the placebo group can be compared.

How to Look at Study Results

There are some important pitfalls to avoid when considering the results of a study.

Is there a statistical difference between the results the groups? If, say, one group of children on amoxicillin took 30 hours for their ear pain to disappear, and the comparison group of children on a new experimental drug took 29.7 hours, there is probably really no difference between the two groups. The numbers may look different, but if they're that close than there really isn't any meaningful difference. Stated more formally, if there is no *statistical* difference between two results, there is no difference at all. See the appendix for more details about making decisions based on medical statistics.

Is there a clinical difference between the results of the groups? This is a very important point that I often see overlooked in newspaper accounts of new medical studies. Let's say the new wonderdrug for asthma helps a patient taking it exhale with 10 percent more force than the older drug. What does that mean? I really have no idea. What I really want to know is: does the new drug help my patient really feel better? Miss fewer days of school? Have stronger lung capacity that allows her to participate in sports? Although measuring how fast you can exhale is important in the research world, in clinical practice I am much more impressed by clinical results that will really make a difference to my patients. This is again especially true when considering a new medicine, with its higher cost and higher risk of unknown side effects. Your attitude toward any new drug should be: prove to me that you're better than what I've already got to justify your cost and risks.

Is there evidence of bias? Is there any reason to suspect the motives of the people running the study? Many drug studies are paid for by pharmaceutical companies that want to make money by selling the drug. If the study is funded by a pharmaceutical company, or if the investigators are employees or consultants of a pharmaceutical company, you need to be mindful that their results could be biased. This doesn't mean that every sponsored study is untrustworthy, just that you need to be aware of who is paying for what. Some positive studies are bound to be from drug companies, but if *all* of the data supporting the use of a drug comes directly from its manufacturer, look out.

Was the study large enough? A study involving 12 kids is much less impressive than a study of 120, which is less impressive than 1,200. The more children involved, the better the chance of seeing a true difference in the result. If there are too few kids involved in a study, you really can't say for sure that the results are valid for a wide and diverse number of children.

Are the results unique and unexpected? Before I change my practices, I like to see multiple studies showing a new product is superior. Don't be fooled by a single groundbreaking study that shows something new. Often results become less impressive when studies are repeated.

MORE ABOUT PLACEBOS AND THE NATURAL HISTORY OF DISEASE

As I've said, any new drug being studied has got to be compared with either a placebo, or if more appropriate some existing standard therapy for the condition. However, you should not assume that the placebo therapy is completely ineffective. In fact, in many cases the placebo effect accounts for more of the improvement than the study drug itself!

Consider the most common reason pediatricians prescribe antibiotics: the ordinary ear infection, or otitis media. In numerous studies repeated in many countries, about 60 percent of children have relief of pain and fever within twenty-four hours of placebo therapy for ear infections. If you wait until two to three days, 80 percent of children treated *without any antibiotics* will have resolution of their symptoms. Studies of antibiotics to treat ear infections show they are effective—just about any antibiotic ever studied increases your chance of successful treatment by 12 percent. After twenty-four hours on placebo, 60 percent of kids feel better, versus 67 percent on antibiotics. In the case of ear infections, the majority of the healing is going to take place with no help at all from the antibiotic; the placebo effect is in fact much larger (60 percent) than the incremental added effectiveness of the antibiotic (12 percent).

There's more to consider when you look at the example of antibiotics for ear infections: they may help prevent rare but serious complications, and they may be more dramatically effective for younger children or for children who are more ill. There are also pitfalls in the diagnosis of ear infections that may make some of the studies less reliable. Nonetheless, therapeutic decisions for common ear infections are an excellent example of how we have come to exaggerate our reliance on medication for a cure, rather than trying to help a child feel better while the body heals itself.

This brings us to a final, astonishing point about the body, the mind, and therapeutics. The assumption in the medical field has always been that a placebo is a placebo. Giving a sugar pill doesn't do anything. It just allows the disease to proceed naturally, as if you did nothing at all. That makes sense, right?

It turns out that a placebo can in fact have significant effects on real, genuine healing. Elegant experiments have been done comparing not a drug versus a placebo, but the same drug given either while the patient is watching the nurse versus surreptitiously. The set up has been replicated under several circumstances, but it basically goes like this: a patient is hooked up to an intravenous line, where a medicine can be administered in full view of the patient or secretly through a remote controlled infusion pump. It's the same medicine, but by giving it in two different ways we can better see how the mind's perception of getting medicine changes the way the medicine works. In several examples of this kind of study, medicines are far more effective if given openly by a nurse than if given secretly. This has been shown not only for medicines that treat subjective complaints such as pain and anxiety, but also for medicines that change simple vital signs like the heart rate.

So the "placebo effect" is more than a "nothing effect"—patients who think they're getting medicine may well improve more than patients who are not treated at all, even if the treatment itself is a sham.

Studies like these illustrate just how complex and powerful the mind can be. Although clinical trials are crucial in the development and study of new medications, often psychological factors may be a tremendous factor in how a patient feels and how a patient responds to medication.

To put this in perspective: when your child is ill, you can think of three components to healing. The first is the natural history of the disease: that is, what would have happened anyway, or what would happen if you did absolutely nothing. The second is the placebo, or mind-body effect: how a child begins to feel better when they know their parents are taking care of them, and how the confidence of their parents helps them improve. The third part of healing is from medical therapeutics: how the doctor's prescribed intervention helps. Only the third component is easily measured by a clinical trial, but all three can be significant ways for your children to become well.

Medical doctors are notoriously suspicious of the placebo effect, and have long equated placebo therapy with shams and quackery. Yet in some cases children treated with placebos can indeed heal nearly as well as those treated with modern medicines. In Chapter 11 we'll look into alternative health providers and alternative health products that exploit psychology far better than medical doctors ever have.

Rigorous clinical trials, well designed and free of bias, are the best way to prove a new medicine is worthwhile. Reading the medical literature to review these studies yourself may seem daunting, and you may wish to rely on your physician to keep up-to-date on this literature rather than doing it yourself. Nonetheless, understanding the design and purpose of clinical trials can help you "read between the lines" like a true insider. In the next section, we'll move beyond the science of studying medicines to learn some insider tips on how to use them best.

THE CARE AND USE OF MEDICINES

Medical doctors use a variety of tools to prevent and treat disease. Counseling about diet and lifestyle can help with many problems, and sometimes listening and encouraging can by themselves be very effective. But what makes medical doctors unique is our training and expertise in prescribing medicines.

Medicines are potent. They can dramatically improve your health. However, they all have potentially serious side effects, and have to be chosen and used with care. An insider's knowledge can reveal some important tips about medicine: how to choose them, use them, and not be abused by them.

Keep in mind that most medicines go by at least two names. The chemical name, which is also called the generic name, is in lower case, and is usually preferred in academic circles. But practicing physicians will often refer to a drug by its brand or trade name, which will be capitalized. For instance, most physicians call a common fever medicine Tylenol, which is more academically known as acetaminophen. To avoid confusion, try to make sure you know both the generic and brand names for all of your medicines.

DECISIONS ABOUT MEDICINES: HOW TO DECIDE WHICH ONE IS YOR YOU

Usually, the doctor chooses the medicine. But with some insider tips, you can help your physician choose a medicine that will be effective without costing you a fortune.

Though your pediatrician would like to choose a good, inexpensive product, keep in find that other forces are at work to influence the decision. Pharmaceutical companies spend billions to promote their products, both to the physicians and directly to parents. Print, television, and Internet advertising saturates many of the resources that doctors rely on for information. Legions of attractive pharmaceutical sales people appear in doctors' offices every day, bearing goodies and food. All of this is geared toward pushing the latest and most expensive medication. Although the pharmaceutical sales people are tightly regulated to prevent mischief, even when all of the regulations are followed they are still going to represent their product in the best possible way. Their singular goal is to increase sales. This may not be to your benefit—a cheaper medicine may be just as good as or better than the latest and most expensive wonderdrug.

What's so special about a prescription medicine anyway? Contrary to popular belief, a prescription medicine is not necessarily "stronger" or less safe than an over-the-counter (OTC) medicine. The decision whether a medicine requires a prescription is not made by the Food and Drug Administration (FDA), but by the company that manufactures the medicine. It is a marketing decision, made to maximize sales and profits.

A "new" medicine may be a lawful copy of a competitor's off-patent product, or a combination of existing medicines, or a genuinely new product. When a company develops any of these to sell, it decides whether to seek approval for the medicine as a prescription or an OTC product. (All new prescription applications and many new OTC applications must have FDA approval before they can be sold. In some cases, OTC medicines that are using well-established ingredients in approved doses can skip the approval process.) In general, the FDA is much more stringent about OTC products. They must be proven to be very safe or have been used for many years to be approved for sale without a prescription. But some extremely safe medicines are submitted for prescription status rather than OTC. For instance, the newer allergy medicines like loratidine (Claritin), or fexofenadine (Allegra) are far safer in many ways than the older allergy medicine diphenhydramine (Benadryl), yet their manufacturers first sought approval as prescription medicines. (At ordinary doses, the newer agents are less sedating, and less likely to cause serious reactions like urinary retention. Following an accidental overdose, the newer drugs are also less likely to cause serious harm.) Perhaps they can sell prescriptions at a higher price, or perhaps prescriptions themselves carry a "magic" quality, seeming more effective than on OTC product. In any case, Claritin is now sold over the counter, having been resubmitted as an OTC product as it drew close to losing its patent. Meanwhile the manufacturer began to sell prescription Clarinex, encouraging physicians to switch over their Claritin patients to this newer drug with more-expensive prescription status. Certainly, both Claritin and Clarinex are both very safe and effective allergy medicines, and they've both helped a lot of people feel better. But keep in mind that decisions about how to market these and other drugs are made by their manufacturers with an eye toward maximizing profit.

By the way, I don't mean to pick on Claritin. There are many other examples of excellent, effective, and safe products being available over the counter that are underused because they lack the prescription cachet and profit margin. Some of them include: ibuprofen (Motrin, Advil), acetaminophen (Tylenol), ranitidine (Zantac), and omeprazole (Prilosec). These are all just as effective as newer "me too" drugs that have replaced their prescription versions. Similarly, the list of prescription cold and cough products is staggering, especially considering that most of them contain the exact same ingredients as over the counter products. They're sold by prescription to seem more magical and effective in the eyes of gullible physicians and patients. With medicines you don't necessarily get more if you pay more.

That leads us to another related question: is it worth it to pay more for a brand name product? In some cases, you don't have a choice—newer products have patent protection, meaning that only the company that owns the product can produce and sell it. But often, as we've seen, the newer product has no important advantages

> ☞ **Choose the medicine that is likely to work the best with the minimum of cost and side effects. Whether it is prescription or nonprescription doesn't matter.**

over the older medicine that may be available in a generic form. In fact, I'd always prefer to use an older drug, as more years of experience with it means I'm more familiar with it and there's less likelihood of a surprise safety concern.

Always choose a generic version if one is available. Brand name products have no advantages, though of course the people who market these products disagree. Though some physicians really do seem to cling to certain brands, there is overwhelming evidence that generic products are just as safe and effective.

> ☞ **Generics are fine.**

One minor caveat might be with certain time release preparations, which may not have exactly the same way of releasing the drug as their brand name versions. If your child depends on a time release product, I'd certainly try the generic first, but you may see a difference compared with a brand name.

In choosing a prescription, many families can pay less if the medication is on their insurance company's formulary. This is a list of drugs that is available at a lower copay to the patient. The list will not necessarily reflect the "best" drugs in a group, only which ones will cost you less. Usually, generic products are automatically available at a low copay. If no generic is available, or if a newer product really is superior, you may want to work with your pharmacist and physician to choose a medicine at the lowest copay. This is especially important if the medicine will need to be taken for a long time. Keep in mind that many medicines are quite similar, and your physician may well be able to choose a very effective medicine that will be cheaper for you. But we pediatricians do not routinely keep lists of these formularies ourselves—they change often, they're different for every insurance plan, and they're one more list that we don't want to worry about. Don't be shy about bringing copies of formulary pages in, or asking your pharmacist to suggest a similar medicine to your physician if it will help you save money.

To summarize: your goal is to choose a medicine that works, is safe, and has less cost.

- DO choose an older medicine or generic product, if available.
- DO consult your insurance company formulary if you must use a brand name product.

- DO NOT be concerned whether the product is by prescription or OTC.
- DO NOT allow advertising to lead the decision.

MEDICINES: HOW TO USE THEM

The most important way to safely and effectively use medicines is to understand and follow the instructions. Doctors won't necessarily make this easy—we mumble, and we write the prescriptions themselves in illegible codes. (They're secret, but I'll tell you them anyway. Some common abbreviations: BID = two times a day; TID = three times a day; QID = four times a day; po = take by mouth; qAC = before meals; qHS = at bedtime; prn = as needed; sig = instructions.) Make sure that you understand exactly what the doses and instructions are for every suggested medicine, both prescription and OTC. Don't assume that the pharmacist can read the prescription correctly.

Medicines will have an expiration date, or maybe more than one. The pharmacist will print a label with an expiration date, usually one year or so after the prescription is filled. This can be helpful, but better than this will be a manufacturer's date stamped on the bottle itself. Rely on the manufacturer's stamp if it is available. Most drugs may lose a little of their potency after that expiration date, but can still be safely taken if needed. (The single exception to this is an older antibiotic called tetracycline, which can actually change to a toxic compound if taken far after its expiration date.) If your child needs to take a medicine long term, check the expiration date before you pay for it. Insiders ask the pharmacist for good fresh stuff if they know they'll need to hold on to the supply for a while.

Some medicines, especially liquid antibiotics, are supposed to be kept refrigerated. For these medicines, a brief stint on the countertop overnight will not harm their potency. They'll certainly be ruined if kept in a hot car. Ask your pharmacist if a medicine really needs to be replaced after exposure to heat.

Many medicines have special instructions regarding their relationship with meals. In most cases these are guidelines that are meant to maximize the effectiveness of the medicine, control the rate at which they're absorbed, or avoid stomach upset. Usually it's better to "bend the rules" a little bit rather than skip a dose entirely if you've forgotten to keep an empty stomach.

One common chronic medical problem in children is asthma, which is usually treated with inhaled medications. It's especially important that you know how to use the devices correctly, and keep them clean and in good working order. Bring these medicines and their delivery devices with you to follow-up visits to make sure you're using them correctly.

AVOID SIDE EFFECTS

By their nature, all medicines are potent biological agents. In addition to their therapeutic effects, every single drug has the potential to cause unwanted effects as well. Some are predictable (Benadryl makes many people drowsy), and some are not (allergic reactions are always possible.) Some occur more frequently if certain drugs are used in combination. Some are common and well known to pediatricians, but some are so rare that your physician may not consider the possibility that your problem is caused by a medicine.

The FDA requires extensive studies of new medicines before they are sold, to document both effectiveness and safety. But potentially serious adverse reactions may not be known until after the medicine is widely used, especially if the side effect is rare. You should be quite suspicious of the potential for side effects if anything unexpected is happening while your child is taking a medicine. This is especially true for newer drugs. You

> If things are not going well, *always* consider if a symptom is being caused by a medicine. Many times I've been able to help by stopping a medicine that was actually making things worse.

or your doctor should report any suspected adverse reaction to the FDA at www.fda.gov/medwatch, so that rare reactions can be tracked and studied. Reporting drug reactions is one of the most important ways to protect patients against uncommon but significant adverse events.

If you suspect an adverse reaction to a medicine, let your doctor know right away. If the reaction is worsening or serious, you should stop the medicine. If it is not too serious, you should talk with your physician before making any changes in your child's therapy.

Make sure your child's physician knows all of the medicines you are taking, including nonprescription products. This helps avoid drug–drug interactions, which can be a serious problem especially if your child has complex needs and is on several medicines. The best way to make sure you communicate this accurately is to bring all of your child's medicines with you to appointments.

Another aspect of medicine safety is keeping children from taking them by accident. If you have toddlers, you need to keep medicines way out of their reach. Childproof caps are important, but a resourceful and determined toddler can get through them quickly. Also, do not refer to medicine or vitamins as "candy" or allow babies to play with medicine containers, even empty ones. You may need to keep prescriptions away from teenagers, too—they can deliberately or accidentally take them incorrectly.

What If My Child Just Won't Take the Medicine?

I've met many children who just absolutely refuse to take medicine. They clamp their mouths shut, they fight, and they spit it back out five minutes later! If this reminds you of your child, these tips can help:

- Avoid giving unnecessary medicines or vitamins. Don't give them more opportunities to practice fighting!
- Always try to get a medicine that tastes good and is given as infrequently as possible, for the fewest possible doses.

- For babies, a device is available that looks like a pacifier with a reservoir inside to deposit liquid medicine behind the tongue where the baby won't taste it. Clever! It works best if your baby is already used to a pacifier.
- Have your child practice taking "medicine" when they're *not* sick. When a child is already miserable with an earache, that's a terrible time to try to get them to accept something they already know they don't like! Practice when your child is in a good mood.
- Practice with something really tasty, like chocolate syrup, peanut butter, or cake frosting—or even a little spoonful of cake decorating jimmies. Be creative! Your child will happily lap these things off of a spoon. Once they're good at that, encourage them to try the same yummy stuff out of a medicine cup or another more "medical" device.
- Once a child will take something tasty out of a medicine cup, *add* that tasty thing to the medicine next time. You should make sure with your pharmacist that mixing food into a medicine is OK, but I can't think of any example where a bit of chocolate syrup mixed into medicine could cause a problem.
- Give your child choices if possible: liquid or chewable? From a cup, spoon, or dosing syringe? Some pharmacies can add one of dozens of flavors to any medicine—let your child choose.
- Remember rewards! If they get it down and keep it down, they get seven M&Ms! (I like a yummy food treat in this case because it will help get rid of the taste; I like a specific counted number of items because counting itself will help with distraction. Do the big countdown of M&Ms before the medicine is taken.)

Medicines are powerful, and when used correctly can greatly improve a child's life and health. Many excellent, safe, and effective medicines are affordable. Some, but not all, adverse reactions can be avoided. Follow the insider tips in this chapter to get the most benefit from your child's medicines without unintentionally harming your child or spending a fortune.

11

ALTERNATIVES TO MEDICINE

Millions of Americans reach beyond their traditional physicians to alternative sources of care. This nontraditional medicine includes an eclectic and diverse collection of methods and philosophies that can be difficult to define as a single group, but seem to share some common elements:

- They have not been proven to be effective by scientific, reproducible, and objective observations.
- They are distrusted and dismissed by medical doctors.
- They are often rooted in "vitalism" or a belief in supernatural forces whose mechanisms defy explanation by current scientific knowledge.

Proponents of alternative medicine have their own viewpoints:

- They do work, but clinical trials don't demonstrate their effectiveness because treatment is not aimed at a measurable endpoint, but rather on overall "wellness." Besides, individualized remedies can't be tested the same way that standardized medicines are.
- Some remedies have been used for thousands of years, and that proves they work.
- Many alternative medicine practitioners don't trust medical doctors and their methods, either.
- Science can only go so far in explaining things. Just because we can't understand it doesn't mean it doesn't work.

In this chapter, we'll take an objective look at alternative medicine. What's the history and rationale behind these methods? Can it help your children stay healthy or recover from illness in a way that's safer than traditional medicine? I'll focus on herbal medicine, homeopathy, and chiropractic, as these are among the most popular and easily accessible forms of alternative care that are used in children.

For clarity, I'm going to use the familiar term "alternative medicine" to collectively refer to these approaches that are generally outside of the mainstream of medicine that is practiced by most doctors. In the medical literature, the most popular name used now is "complementary and alternative medicine", often abbreviated as "CAM." Other terms used are integrative medicine, holistic medicine, or unorthodox medicine. The phrase "allopathic medicine" is sometimes used to refer to the traditional or "standard" medicine practiced by most physicians. Traditional physicians themselves are either "Medical Doctors" (MDs) or "Doctors of Osteopathy" (DOs). Although most medical schools confer the "MD" degree, graduates from a smaller number of institutions get a "DO" after their name. Philosophically, osteopaths feel that they treat "the whole person" rather than symptoms. Practically speaking, osteopathic physicians are licensed to prescribe medicine and perform surgery just as MDs do, and most DOs practice medicine in a manner very similar to MDs.

HERBS AND SUPPLEMENTS

Herbal medicine encompasses the use of plant, fungal, and soil-based material to promote health and treat disease. Many human cultures have relied on these sorts of remedies for millennia, finding unique health benefits in things found in their local environments. Many plant extracts have been found to have potent and useful medical properties:

- Digitalis (Foxglove) can be used to treat heart failure.
- Aspirin was originally derived from the bark of a willow tree.
- The modern cancer treating medicine Taxol comes from a yew tree.

Natural plant materials may certainly have health benefits, in the same way that purified chemical pharmaceutical agents may also have medical properties. However, the legal and research atmosphere surrounding herbal products makes using them different from using medications.

All medicines marketed in the United States are required to have their safety and effectiveness demonstrated to the Food and Drug Administration (FDA) *before* they can be sold. Herbal products and dietary supplements are regulated differently—as long as they don't make claims that they are medicines, they can be freely sold and marketed without FDA approval. In fact, unless evidence arises that the product is actually dangerous, herbs and supplements are not monitored in any way by the government. It is rare that enough evidence of harm accumulates for the FDA to ban an herbal ingredient, but occasionally products with lead contamination or unsafe ingredients such as ephedra have been taken off the market. Many herbal products are labeled that they "are not intended to cure, treat, or diagnose any disease." This statement counterbalances any vague health-related claims on the packaging, so the supplement can be sold with looser regulatory oversight.

Though products marketed as supplements cannot make specific health claims on their labeling, the supplement industry has found plenty of ways to convince the public of their health benefits indirectly. Ingredients and formulas can be promoted through books, lectures, speakers, newsletters, "info-mercial" broadcasts, Internet sites, and claims made by salespeople at the stores. None of these venues are adequately monitored by the FDA or any other authority to ensure that claims of effectiveness or safety are accurate.

In addition, the FDA requires that medicines have proven purity and consistency: what it says on the label must be what is in the bottle. No legal regulations guarantee the purity or potency of herbal products. Many herbal manufacturers participate in voluntary programs that allow a quality seal to be printed on the label if certain standard measurements of purity are met. Seals that attest to purity include "USP," "Good Housekeeping," "Consumer-Lab.com," and "NSF International." None of these organizations are obligated by law to report or investigate untrue claims, and each sets up their own rules of testing in order to print their seal. Still, participation in one of these plans is better than nothing if you are looking to guarantee that what you're buying is what you expect.

Relatively few herbal products have been tested for effectiveness using the "gold standard" applied to medicines. A "double-blinded clinical trial" requires that a group of patients with the same problem be divided randomly into two groups, one of which receives the drug while the other half receives a placebo (for details see Chapter 10). To prove that a medicine or herb is effective, it must help the people who receive the drug more that the volunteers who received placebo. Though all medicines (except some very old ones that were "grandfathered") have met this standard of proof, very few herbs have been tested with this degree of vigor. Even fewer have been tested for effectiveness or safety in children.

The following is a list of common herbal products that have been suggested for use in chil-

> ☞ **Neither the FDA nor any other government authority regulates the content, purity, safety, or effectiveness of any herbal product.**

dren. I've tried to cover herbal products that have been studied with the most rigor, either in children or adults, and I've stressed both products that have been shown to be helpful along with products that are potentially harmful and should be avoided.

Aloe Vera

A gel from the leaves of the aloe plant can be used as a salve for sunburns and other skin irritations. Animal and laboratory-based studies have shown it has antibiotic properties and can speed wound healing, confirmed by at least one study in adult volunteers. Rare, mild skin allergies have been reported. Serious gastrointestinal problems can be triggered if aloe vera is swallowed.

Bee Pollen

This natural product is touted to treat allergic diseases including asthma and hay fever. There is no evidence that it works, and it has triggered fatal allergic reactions. It should not be used.

Calendula

Appearing in teas, salves, cosmetics, and other preparations for topical use, calendula may act to help wound healing and prevent infection. No studies have evaluated calendula for safety or effectiveness in children, but it has been widely used for centuries and is probably safe.

Chamomile

Chamomile tea is a very commonly used herbal preparation. One study did show chamomile (combined with several other herbs) to be more effective than placebo in calming infants with colic-like symptoms. It has also been touted to help with abdominal pain, insomnia, or anxiety in older children—though there are no studies confirming these effects. Other than rare allergic reactions, chamomile appears to cause minimal side effects or drug interactions. Chamomile can also be used topically, and laboratory studies have shown it to have antibacterial properties. However, studies in humans (which have never included children) have shown inconsistent effectiveness for topical chamomile as an agent to improve wound healing.

Echinacea

Initial studies in adults showed promise for echinacea to reduce the severity and duration of the common cold. However, better studies performed in follow-up failed to confirm that echinacea preparations really made any difference. Studies in children have not shown effectiveness either. Though allergic reactions are possible, echinacea appears to be quite safe. Chizukit—a combination of echinacea, vitamin C, and a natural bee resin—is marketed in Israel. Though many children were unable to take Chizukit because of the taste, children who were able to tolerate this preparation did have fewer respiratory infections than children given an equally bad-tasting placebo. Combinations of echinacea with other products have also shown at least modest benefits as cold prevention or treatment options.

Evening Primrose Oil

Taken orally for a wide variety of ailments, evening primrose oil in children has been best studied as part of a regimen for treating eczema. Several studies have shown at least modest effectiveness when taken long-term, with minimal side effects.

Fennel

Often prepared medicinally as an extracted oil, fennel is a safe product found in many kitchens. Two studies have shown fennel preparations to be more effective than placebo in reducing fussy symptoms in infants. However, the large volume of tea required in one of the studies could potentially interfere with the baby's consumption of more nutritious milk.

Ginger

This is another common kitchen ingredient that is likely safe for everyone. It has been suggested to treat nausea and other gastrointestinal ailments, and one very small study showed that ginger was effective for nausea associated with motion sickness in children.

Gripe Water

This is not a single product, but rather one of many available different preparations suggested as treatments for fussy infants. Unlike the original formulation, most modern versions do not contain alcohol, but rather are made using miniscule amounts of their active biologic ingredients—in other words, gripe water is now a homeopathic product, quite unlike what was used in prior generations. No good clinical studies of gripe water have been performed.

Herbal Ear Drops

A variety of preparations containing multiple ingredients have been studied. As a group, these preparations may be as effective as medicinal numbing ear drops in reducing the symptoms of an ear infection, though they have not been compared to oral acetaminophen (Tylenol) or watchful waiting. No studies suggest that children who receive these drops recover from their infection faster than children who receive nothing at all.

Kava Kava

This herb has been suggested to help with sleep problems, but it can rarely cause potentially deadly liver damage. Because of safety concerns, kava kava should not be used in children.

Melatonin

A natural human hormone, melatonin has been studied to help children with developmental problems achieve regular sleep–wake cycles. It may be helpful in older children with trouble falling asleep, or to help offset the effects of jet lag. In children with preexisting epilepsy, melatonin can increase seizure activity. Reports of adverse effects in otherwise healthy children are very rare, but minimal studies have been performed in preschoolers.

Peppermint Oil

A well-designed but short-term study of peppermint oil in older children suffering from chronic abdominal pain showed a beneficial effect of enteric-coated peppermint oil capsules. It may not be possible for preschoolers to swallow this sort of capsule whole, and unfortunately uncoated peppermint oil can be irritating. Still, this promising study confirms that this otherwise safe product may be quite helpful for some children.

Probiotics

The use of collections of "friendly" bacteria has been suggested to prevent or treat a variety of problems, including allergic diseases, diarrhea, and irritable bowel syndrome. There is excellent evidence that probiotic supplements can shorten the course of common viral diarrheal illnesses, and can probably prevent antibiotic-associated diarrhea as well. Because they are live bacterial products, they should be used with caution in children with poor immune systems, including premature babies. Probiotic bacteria are available from food sources (yogurt, kefir, or miso) or from medicinal supplements (Culturelle, Lactinex, or other brands). Lactobacillus or Bifidobacterium are the most well-studied probiotic bacterial species groups.

Psyllium

Ground psyllium seed is an effective bulking laxative, though it must be taken with plenty of water. Fiber laxatives, whether medically packaged (Metamucil) or "natural," can worsen constipation if taken without enough water.

Riboflavin

Also known as vitamin B_2, riboflavin in relatively high doses has been shown in well-designed adult studies to be effective in preventing migraine headaches; in fact, it may be as effective as some commonly used medications, with far fewer side effects. A safe and effective dose for children has not been established. If your child has migraine headaches, speak with a neurologist or pediatrician about the latest information on the possible role of riboflavin as well as other "alternative" methods (acupuncture, massage, and biofeedback), nonmedical approaches (identification and avoidance of triggers), and medicines for prevention and treatment.

Star Anise

Given as an herbal tea to treat fussy infants, star anise can cause neurologic problems. European reports have suggested that some star anise preparations have been contaminated with related species that are even more toxic. Because of these safety concerns, star anise should not be used in children.

Tea Tree Oil

This product has antibiotic and antifungal properties, and has been suggested to treat cradle cap and minor skin infections in toddlers and babies. When used topically, rare but potentially serious allergic reactions have been reported, along with local irritation if used full strength on broken skin. Tea tree oil can cause confusion and stupor in toddlers if taken orally. No good studies confirming the effectiveness of tea tree oil for any condition in young children have been reported.

Valerian Root

There are several good studies in adults supporting the use of valerian as a sleep aid, which unlike some medicines for insomnia does not seem to cause any morning "hangover" effect. It can impair driving skills in adults and regular use of higher doses may lead to withdrawal symptoms if the product is stopped abruptly. Though no studies have looked at the use of valerian in preschoolers, it is marketed both alone and in combination with a variety of other herbs as a calming or relaxing supplement.

Vitamin C (Ascorbic Acid)

Vitamin C is essential to good health. In fact, lack of this nutrient historically caused the death of more sailors than pirates, wars, and storms combined. Though people lacking in dietary vitamin C can become quite ill, ordinary foods contain enough vitamin C that clinical signs of deficiency are very rarely seen in the developed world. Though touted to prevent the common cold, regular doses of vitamin C have been shown to be ineffective in preventing or ameliorating colds in children. So-called megadoses (more than 500 mg per day in preschoolers) are also ineffective, and may cause kidney damage.

Vitamins (Multivitamins)

Vitamins are necessary for good health, and their "minimum daily requirements" are usually met by an ordinary diet that in the United States includes enriched grains. If your child is a picky eater, it makes sense to give a multivitamin to "cover all of the bases." However, extra-high doses of vitamins are at best a waste of money and at worst toxic. It also makes no sense to spend extra for high priced proprietary or "natural" types of vitamin extracts. To your child's body, vitamins are the same no matter what the source. Use an inexpensive generic multivitamin, preferably chewable once the child is old enough to handle that. Don't refer to them as candy or in any way encourage your child to take "extras"—as with all medicines, multivitamins need to be stored safely away from young children.

Zinc

As with vitamin C, zinc is a required nutrient, and lack of zinc may indeed cause important health problems. The question is, does *extra* zinc improve the health of people who already have adequate zinc in their diet, as do most people in the developed world? Though never studied in preschool-age children, the best controlled studies done in older children and adolescents showed no effect of zinc lozenges in helping children recover faster from a cold. In addition, the lozenges themselves occasionally caused side effects including nausea and oral discomfort.

Using Herbs Wisely

If you choose to try herbal products, keep these tips in mind:

- Herbal products may indeed have potent biologic properties. As with any biologic agents that have an effect on your child's body, side effects are possible. No product can at the same time have a biologic effect yet be completely safe for everyone. Beware of unreasonable claims as to the safety of herbal products. There is no reason to think that something that claims to be "natural" is automatically safer than a medicine.
- Likewise, be wary of unreasonable claims of the effectiveness of an herbal remedy. It is unlikely that any single product can cure a wide variety of ailments.
- Buy from an established store that is more likely to purchase through well-established distributors. Look for freshness dates and be suspicious of packaging that may not have been stored well.
- Herbal products may interact with traditional medicines. Some of these interactions are known and predictable, but if your child is taking multiple medications the risk of seeing an unexpected interaction increases dramatically.
- Be extremely cautious when considering the use of an herbal product manufactured outside of the United States or Europe. Though most European countries regulate herbal products more tightly than we do, herbs from other parts of the world have sometimes been found to be contaminated with toxins, heavy metals, or unexpected potent medications.
- The strength and potency of herbal products can very widely between brands. Though there's no guarantee that what's on the label accurately reflects what's in the bottle, you should try to compare fixed measurable strengths like "milligrams" between brands and manufacturers.
- Pregnant women should be *very* cautious about taking any biologic agent, including any medicine or herbal product.

HOMEOPATHY

Unlike herbal products and supplements, homeopathic remedies do not use biologic agents as active chemicals. Homeopathy does not rely on chemistry or physical laws to explain how its treatments work, but rather on "healing energy" conferred to the homeopathic product through the super-dilution of a noxious or poisonous agent.

Homeopathy was invented by a German physician, Samuel Hahnemann (1755–1843), who saw how misguided the mainstream medical practices of his day had become. Bloodletting, purging, and other quackery were the main treatments offered by most physicians, and they did far more harm than good. The thinking by most physicians of that time was that illness was caused by an imbalance of body humors that had to be treated by rebalancing the humors in the opposite direction. For instance, fever was treated by removing the "hot" humor of blood. Realizing that this philosophy was misguided and giving rise to harmful "treatments," Hahnemann devised a new theory, the "law of similars." He thought that symptoms could be relieved by giving the patient very small amounts of an agent that caused similar symptoms when given in larger amounts to his volunteers. In a process called "proving," Hahnemann gave extracts of plants and other products to volunteers and recorded their symptoms. When he discovered, for instance, that a certain plant *caused* stomach upset, he reasoned that an extremely diluted sample of that same plant could *cure* an upset stomach in another patient. Furthermore, he proposed that the more diluted the preparation of that plant was, the more powerful the agent became in reducing those symptoms. This became known as the "law of infinitesimals." It is of course the opposite of the ordinary dose–response relationship expected of medicines, where higher doses achieve stronger results.

Homeopathic remedies were far safer than what medical doctors were doing in the nineteenth century, and became popular among many medical practitioners. At the turn of the twentieth century, there were twenty-two dedicated homeopathic medical schools in the United States. All were closed by 1930, as medical education advanced and began to rely more on scientific inquiry and provable theories.

To make a homeopathic remedy, the original substance is crushed or mixed with water or alcohol. It is then repeatedly diluted 1:10 or 1:100 times, with vigorous shaking ("succession") between each step. On the label of a homeopathic product, a capital X means a 1/10 dilution, and a multiplier in front of the X means how many times that 1:10 dilution was performed. Thus, a 3X product is diluted to 1/1000. The letter "C" means a 1/100 dilution, so that a "3C" product is diluted to one in one million parts. As the law of infinitesimals means that the more dilutions, the stronger the agent, some of the "strongest" homeopathic remedies are made at 30C strength—that's diluted to 1 followed by 60 zeros.

Hahnemann himself realized that with extreme dilutions, no amount of the original substance would actually still be contained in his remedies. He felt that the medicinal effect was not conferred by the agent itself, but by a "spirit-like" property left behind.

Thus, homeopathic remedies are very distinct from herbal products, and these should not be lumped together. Unlike herbal remedies, homeopathy relies on a mystical, unproven mechanism that contradicts what is understood about chemistry and biology. Although there have been isolated cases of contaminated homeopathic products causing potential harm, by their very nature correctly prepared homeopathic remedies are themselves harmless, as they are entirely inert.

Despite widespread international use, there is no evidence supporting the clinical effectiveness of any homeopathic product in children. The only well-designed, blinded trial of homeopathy that has been published in a widely distributed journal was unable to show that individualized homeopathic remedies were better than placebo in hastening the resolution of an ear infection. The vast majority of homeopathic products have never been studied in any objective or reproducible manner.

The bottom line with homeopathic remedies: they probably won't do any harm, as long as use of these products doesn't take the place of proven therapies for treatable conditions. But there is no evidence that they're effective, nor any logical reason to think that they ought to work.

CHIROPRACTIC

Daniel David Palmer, a grocer with experience in magnetic and other meta-physical healing methods, founded chiropractic in 1895. His theory was that all human diseases were caused by blockages to the flow of nerve signals. Most of these blockages were caused by "subluxations" in the spine, which could be corrected by external manipulation. Once these subluxations were fixed, the body would heal itself through the flow of an "innate life force" to the affected organs.

Medical doctors use the term subluxation to mean a physical misalignment of bones, where one surface doesn't fit against the next bone correctly, as if ice cream were falling off of a cone. Medical subluxations are always visible on x-rays, and cause pain and distortion of function from the physical change in the ways the bones are touching. In contrast, chiropractic subluxations are a conceptualization rather than a physical relationship between bones. They cannot be specifically demonstrated on x-rays, and are not diagnosed identically by different chiropractors.

There is controversy about subluxations and the appropriate scope of chiro-practic therapy within the chiropractic community. A minority of chiropractors reject Palmer's theory of subluxations entirely, and many of these practitioners limit their practice to treating musculoskeletal complaints. On the other end of the spectrum are so-called "straight" chiropractors, who feel that all human ailments are from spinal subluxations that need to be treated in everyone. In the middle ground are "mixers" who use traditional chiropractic spinal manip-ulation in addition to massage therapy, nutritional advice, or a great variety of other diagnostic and treatment modalities to treat and prevent disease. This term is used derisively by "straight" chiropractors to refer to those who mix in other treatment modalities, and is not accepted by the mixers.

Palmer's proposed mechanism by which chiropractic heals or prevents dis-ease has not withstood scientific scrutiny. To be sure, nerves that are physically pinched by bones in the spine lead to symptoms including pain and altered sensations, numbness, or tingling. Medical doctors and chiropractors also agree that damaged or pinched nerves can also cause decreased muscle strength and difficulties with motor function. However, there is no proof of an "innate life force" that is supplied by the nerves to *all* of the body's organs, or that interruptions in the functioning of nerves are the root cause of *all* human disease. Furthermore, there is no evidence that chiropractic manipulation alters the flow of information through nerve tissue. Excellent, validated instruments are now available that can test nerve function, looking at nerve impulses with great sensitivity. Though these instruments could be applied to chiropractic studies to measure how adjustments change nerve function, no such studies have been forthcoming.

There is good evidence that chiropractic spinal manipulation can help with some musculoskeletal complaints, as can physical therapy or massage. There is no reliable evidence that chiropractic therapy can treat or prevent other ailments such as allergies, ear infections, colic, or bedwetting. As with homeopathic medicine, chiropractic techniques have seldom been studied in a rigorous scientific fashion, but a few studies have tried to compare chiropractic with standard remedies. Published studies have failed to find any benefit to chiropractic therapy in the treatment of colic, scoliosis, hypertension, tension headaches, or asthma.

Is chiropractic therapy safe? For the most part, yes. Ordinary manipulation has a very low risk, though manipulation of the neck, performed rarely in children, has caused strokes and paralysis. The most risky aspect of chiropractic is the potential to miss or delay the diagnosis of a condition that requires medical therapy. Though chiropractors should be trained to recognize and refer significant medical problems to medical doctors, medical referrals from chiropractors are rare. Many malpractice cases against chiropractors are for complications arising from a delay in the diagnosis of a medical condition.

If you do wish to pursue chiropractic therapy for your children, the following tips can help you choose and work with a good chiropractor:

- Avoid relying on a chiropractor for the *diagnosis* of back pain. As back pain is an uncommon problem in children, when it does occur it is far more likely to herald a significant medical problem than does back pain in adults. Work with your pediatrician or orthopedist to make sure that an urgent medical problem doesn't need to be addressed.
- Avoid chiropractors who offer free x-rays, or who want to perform x-rays on everyone. These studies are not necessary and expose your child to ionizing radiation. Unfortunately, "free x-rays" will invariably lead to finding problems that need to be treated, whether or not they have anything to do with your child's symptoms.
- Chiropractors who advertise "free spinal exams for children" will likewise almost always find "subluxations" that need therapy. Chiropractors may be able to help with specific musculoskeletal complaints, but there is no reason to think that a child who is free of symptoms needs chiropractic therapy.

- Steer clear of chiropractors who push expensive nutritional supplements, homeopathic remedies, or herbal products.
- Do not continue a program of spinal manipulation if you don't see an improvement in symptoms within several weeks; if pain increases, stop immediately.

ALTERNATIVE VERSUS TRADITIONAL MEDICINE

The Maturing of Ideas

In about AD 130, during the Roman Empire, Galen taught that disease was caused by an imbalance of the four body humors blood, phlegm, choler (yellow bile), and melancholy (black bile). A cult-like dogma arose from these principles, and persisted well into the nineteenth century. The idea of balancing and restoring body humors was the basis for obviously harmful therapies like bloodletting and purging, and an almost fanatical devotion to these mystic forces delayed by centuries the adoption of methods and ideas that could genuinely heal. Though it was a slow process, medical doctors eventually came to believe as a profession that a better understanding of the human body was necessary to find better cures. In the twentieth century, scientific observations finally overtook cultism as the basis of medical thought. Rather than base therapy on unproven (and unprovable) ideas, physicians began to examine their patients to discover the underlying basis of disease using the best available technology. Once the true cause of illness is known, treatments can be formulated and then objectively tested. Our understanding of health and disease will continue to evolve and improve through scientific inquiry. Choosing which therapies are best in an ever-evolving field requires objective, measurable proof.

Of the three alternative medicine methods explored in this chapter, herbal products have the best potential to meet this standard, becoming more useful and dependable with further study. Clearly, some herbal products have potent biologic properties, and their chemical constituents can be analyzed and understood. Though there are problems with standardization and regulation, these could be overcome. If proponents of herbal products would embrace the need for controlled clinical trials to prove which herbs work reliably and safely, these products could become an important part of our healing armamentarium. Though some herbs have been studied in this way, there is much to be learned about most herbal remedies.

On the other end of the spectrum, the mechanism through which homeopathic products might improve health is nonsensical. No single homeopathic product has ever been shown to be effective. By lumping homeopathy with other healing methods that show more promise, alternative health proponents do themselves and their patients a disservice. An uncritical acceptance of any and all healing ideas—without any proof of effectiveness or any reliance on mechanisms that make scientific sense—unfortunately characterizes much of the alternative health marketplace.

Chiropractors are in the middle. A minority are insisting that their profession move beyond the dogma of Palmer's subluxations, and use scientific inquiry to evaluate whether their methods work. (The National Association for Chiropractic Medicine and the Canadian Academy of Manipulative Therapists both espouse a more evidence-based view of spinal manipulation.) They are looking to define exactly what problems are best suited to chiropractic care, and what issues are beyond the scope of their skills and training. These chiropractors may well become the future of their profession. However, their numbers are currently outweighed by their colleagues who believe that Palmer's subluxations cause all disease, and that spinal manipulation is the only intervention needed to cure or prevent every malady. Many chiropractors have businesses entangled with other unproven therapies, selling homeopathic and questionable nutritional supplements alongside magnetic healing devices or other chicanery. As medical doctors were finally able to abandon their devotion to the four body humors, chiropractors need to move beyond their commitment to Palmer's original theories in order to find the best way for their methods to genuinely help the most people.

Risks versus Benefits

Even hard-core skeptics of alternative medicines will admit that in most cases therapies from the world of alternative medicine are harmless. It is true that in some isolated cases chiropractic therapy or herbal products have led to genuine injury, but these cases are far outweighed by the hundreds of harmful medical mistakes occurring each day. On balance, is it reasonable that families wish to explore alternative therapies?

A central tenet of deciding whether a therapy is worth pursuing is balancing the potential risk versus the potential benefit. A therapy that is quite risky might be worth trying if the potential benefit is very large. Think about these examples:

1. A fifteen-month-old baby has leukemia. We know that the combination of chemotherapy and radiation used to treat leukemia has tremendous risks, including damage to the heart and lungs, and an increased risk of future cancer. But the potential benefit is that the baby's life can be saved. In this case, even very risky therapy is justified. If it helps, that is wonderful. If it doesn't, the cold truth is that the baby was going to die anyway.

2. A three-week-old baby is fussy. A thorough history and exam has shown that the baby is physically fine and growing, but his fussiness is stressful to his parents. His pediatrician suggests trying Mylicon for "gas." Though Mylicon has never been shown to be beneficial in reducing crying, we know in fact that it is a very safe agent that is nearly free of side effects. Therefore, though the potential benefit is small or nonexistent, the low risk means it might be worth a try. If it helps, great! If not, it was unlikely to do any physical harm.

3. A two-year-old child has a cold. He is a little fussy. His mom buys an over-the-counter homeopathic zinc nasal spray, which seem to help him feel better.

Though she knows that controlled studies really haven't shown that zinc at the dose in this spray is likely to help, she also knows that as a homeopathic product it is very unlikely to cause any harm.

4. Eleven-year-old Betty has recently been diagnosed with diabetes. Instead of taking insulin shots as suggested by her pediatrician and endocrinologist, the child is taken to an alternative therapy center overseas. In addition to the considerable expense, the family endures three weeks of "tests" and "procedures." Upon their return, the child has lost ten pounds. Two years later Betty returns to her pediatrician with continued poor weight gain and now cognitive slowing. Her parents reluctantly begin conventional therapy with insulin for diabetes.

Case (1) is presented in a coldhearted manner, but shows that risks can be justified by a need to treat a deadly illness. Case (2) illustrates that medical doctors can effectively suggest harmless placebos, too. Case (3) may make physicians squirm, but I would suggest that mom's decision is not too different from what was suggested in case (2), that is, to treat a mild illness choose something that you know is safe. It is case (4) that really worries doctors like me.

In case (4), Betty has a serious condition that can lead to death. Though treatment for diabetes can seem discouraging—it is lifelong and involves needles—it very effectively decreases the potential complications of childhood diabetes. The family in this case chose unproven therapy because they were afraid of the risks of conventional therapy, but in doing so they exposed their child to the very real and known risks of not treating her serious condition at all.

MEDICAL DOCTORS AND QUACKERY TODAY

In this chapter I've reviewed the history and methods of some kinds of alternative or nonconventional therapies, pointing out that much of the culture and practice of these methods is intertwined with quackery. That is, unproven or disproven therapies are used without critical and reproducible proof of effectiveness. The modern medical establishment has been dismissive of these therapies, in part because they often don't hold up to scientific scrutiny. The sad truth is that there is plenty of quackery being practiced by medical doctors, too.

Consider some of the disproven therapies that are dispensed every day by medical doctors. We know that the vast majority of cough and congestion illnesses are caused by viruses, and yet a useless antibiotic is prescribed at well over 50 percent of office visits by adults to medical doctors for these complaints. We also know that most over-the-counter and prescription cold medicines prescribed by doctors are completely useless. Doctors will often say that "not enough good studies have been done" to disprove their favorite therapies, but even with clear and convincing evidence many physicians are reluctant to change their habits. It has been shown in numerous studies that diarrhea improves most rapidly with an ordinary diet, yet many pediatricians still suggest a bland, starchy diet for this common condition. Why? Because we *always* have.

Alternative therapy should be held to the same standards expected of conventional medicine: well-designed, double-blinded trials should show that they work before these therapies are encouraged and sold. But we medical doctors need to keep in mind that our own practice often falls short of this goal. Our understanding of health and disease will continue to grow as science evolves. To genuinely help people stay healthy, doctors need to look critically at all aspects of healthcare to ensure that our practices continue to match the best of current knowledge.

ALTERNATIVE MEDICINE: THE COSTS

Though most realms of alternative medicine are safe, they can be expensive. Herbs can be purchased cheaply, but individual consultation with a homeopathic or naturalistic practitioner is pricey. Chiropractic therapy entails ongoing visits and ongoing expense. Consider the costs of these services in addition to their risk: benefit ratio when deciding whether this is how you want to spend your money.

HOW TO USE ALTERNATIVE MEDICINE: AN INSIDER'S ADVICE

First, start with the diagnosis. Medical doctors are the best trained professionals to rely on to determine what might be wrong with your child. We spend far longer in academic and clinical rotations than do any alternative health providers, and our professional boards require ongoing continuing education to keep our skills sharp. Also, only medical doctors do clinical rotations through specialty clinics and hospitals, where we are likely to see the sickest patients. It is those rare cases of serious illness that you are counting on your pediatrician to sniff out, and it is very unlikely that an alternative provider has had the experience or training to recognize or even be aware of rare and serious conditions. Pediatricians are also well-trained to perform ongoing health maintenance visits, using additional historical questions, a comprehensive exam, and focused tests to screen for significant health issues before they become problems.

If your trusted pediatrician suggests a diagnosis that is serious, I would urge you to continue therapy along the lines of the best medical evidence with your pediatrician. By serious, I mean any diagnosis that can lead to harm. This could mean an infection that can cause death (pneumonia), a chronic illness that can affect growth (hypothyroidism), a condition that can make it difficult to succeed in school (dyslexia), or a condition that can lead to depression and social withdrawal (parental divorce). A diagnosis can be entirely behavioral or developmental, and still be serious; though you might not think of these as "medical" diagnoses, your pediatrician's office is still the best place to go for guidance on therapy of *any* condition that can harm your child.

But for most problems that are diagnosed by a pediatrician, the natural history is far more benign. That is, most of the kids I see will get better on their own, sometimes helped by safe and inexpensive symptomatic therapy. Once you've established that your child is at low risk for serious problems, look for therapies that help your child feel better with a low potential for side effects. These might include suggestions from your medical doctor, or perhaps safe treatments from the realm of alternative medicine. And don't dismiss the healing powers of love and affection, which cost nothing at all.

> ☞ **Your pediatrician should make sure your child does not have a dangerous illness before you rely on unproven therapies.**

Parents want to keep their children healthy. Fortunately, many of the most serious health problems that have harmed children in the past are now essentially gone from the developed world. Clean water, adequate nutrition, safer transportation, and vaccines have all but eliminated many of the most deadly problems. But if your child might have a serious health concern, rely on your pediatrician as the best resource for diagnosis and treatment. Many alternative therapies are safe, but have unproven effectiveness. You cannot trust them if your child is truly ill.

If you'd like to find out more about alternative therapies—or more about conventional medicine, for that matter—you'll find internet and other media outlets overflowing with information. Unfortunately, most of what you'll find is unreliable or deliberately misleading. In the next chapter, you'll learn the best ways to do your own research on medical topics: how to find what you need to know while avoiding sources of misinformation that can waste your time.

12

How to Get Reliable Health Information from the Media

Health care information used to be closely guarded by doctors and professional societies. Prevailing wisdom held that people didn't need to know—or want to know—what was going on inside their bodies, and would trust the experts to make the best decisions for them. Physicians acted like parents, making their own decisions and essentially treating their patients like children. Some families may still prefer a so-called "paternalistic" physician, who just tells you exactly what you need to do.

Today, most families wish to be more informed about health care issues. They still may want the experience and perspective of a physician's guidance, but view health care decisions as a collaboration of what they know and what their physician teaches them.

To be effective partners in making health care decisions, parents have to find reliable sources of health care information. Finding information itself isn't difficult—we're awash in information from the print media, TV, and the Internet. The difficulty is separating the good from the bad, the balanced from the biased, and the voices that are trying to teach from the voices that are trying to sell. Health care information is a wild and wooly frontier, as lawless and unregulated as the Old West. With a few minutes and a computer you can find comprehensive health information that would have taken weeks to research fifteen years ago, but you can also find snake-oil salesmen and agenda-driven malcontents who are all too happy to lure you with viciously misguiding information.

You have to watch out, and you have to know whom to believe.

THE TRADITIONAL MEDIA

Newspapers, TV, and radio make up the "traditional media," and remain an important source of health care information for many families. Keep in mind that for the most part these sources are driven by circulation or ratings.

The goal of their programming is to keep you entertained while reading or listening to their product so you'll pay attention to the advertisements. These media outlets tend to oversimplify health stories for maximum "punch." It is more difficult to keep up interest in a long story, so traditional media tends to get the most catchy and provocative information out quickly, with minimal time for elaboration or follow-up.

In 2005, the American Academy of Pediatrics (AAP) updated its policy statement on Sudden Infant Death Syndrome (SIDS). A public health initiative encouraging parents to place babies to sleep on their backs had already led to a 50 percent drop in mortality from SIDS. In this updated statement, eleven specific recommendations were made. But the headlines in American newspapers uniformly stressed only one: pediatricians were now recommending pacifiers. This was in fact an oversimplification; the statement recommended that parents "consider" offering a pacifier at sleep time, with several caveats and qualifiers. From a public health point of view, stronger recommendations were made for several other points: a back-only position is safest for putting your baby down to sleep; sleep surfaces should be firm; soft objects and pillows are dangerous; smoking should be avoided during and after pregnancy; babies should sleep separately but close to their parents; overheating must be avoided; and commercial devices to prevent or provide early warnings about SIDS are discouraged. Several recommendations were also made to avoid the flattening of heads that occasionally occurs with back-sleeping. The statement also made the point that the rate of SIDS among African-Americans remains about double that of Caucasian babies, in part because African-American parents are still twice as likely to put their babies down on their tummies to sleep. There is a good deal of useful information in this 2005 statement, and better public awareness of these issues particularly among the hardest-hit ethnic groups could have a significant impact on children's lives. Yet, the traditional media stressed only a small part of the recommendations, distracting from the most important message.

A surprising inside fact about news and print media information is that these outlets often get "teaser" stories before your doctor will have access to them. Major medical journals provide articles to the science or health editors of news outlets several days before they're published and available for physicians to review. You'll often see stories about the latest "breakthrough" before it is even possible for genuine health authorities to review or respond to the information. Of course once the media's report is out there, the genie is out of the bottle.

It's much more difficult to refute or give balance to a story that's already been percolating in the public. Often, by the time your doctor has had time to review the most recent breakthrough study, the media has moved on to something else.

The traditional media can still be a good source of information as a starting point for your research. More in-depth information can be found through the library and Internet.

> ☞ **Consider health information from traditional media as entertainment only. Look elsewhere for balanced and complete information.**

INFORMATION FROM ADVERTISING

Advertisers are selling things, and any information from a commercial interest that makes money off sales is going to be skewed to put their product in the most positive light.

In the United States, the Federal Trade Commission (FTC) has broad power to regulate consumer advertising. By federal law, advertisements cannot include information that is untrue; they also cannot include information that hasn't been proven to be true, even if later on this information turns out to be factually correct. That is, the makers of a new headache drug can't claim that most people prefer their product unless they've actually surveyed a group of people and can substantiate this claim. Enforcement of federal false advertising laws either occurs through the FTC or through private individuals suing companies for false advertising practices. Many states also have further laws against deceptive advertising practices. However, enforcement of these laws is incomplete. Smaller companies are especially adept at stretching the truth before attracting the attention of enforcement authorities.

Advertisements about medicines, but not herbal products and supplements, are further regulated by the Food and Drug Administration (FDA). If an advertisement mentions the name of a medicine, it must include information about what conditions it is used for and side effects that may occur. Print advertisements in particular have numerous regulations about the size of the type used for the name of the product and other information. Any claims made in the advertisement must be fully supported and endorsed in the official "product insert" approved by the FDA. The FDA actively examines medication advertisements, and often forces drug companies to correct ads to clarify information. Again, this sort of enforcement only applies to medicines; that's why so many alternative health products have an explicit statement that "This product is not intended to diagnose or treat any disease." A statement such as this acts like garlic keeping away a vampire: with this verbiage, the government doesn't consider the product a drug, and can't apply the more stringent rules of drug advertising.

Is It a Drug or Not?

What would you think of a product that said it was used to:

- Improve focus and ability to concentrate
- Increase attention span
- Boost memory functioning
- Increase motivation and energy levels
- Increase study skills
- Boost immune functioning and protect against illness

This is from the advertising material for a widely-sold herbal product for Attention Deficit Disorder (ADD). Below these claims are an extensive section about the symptoms of ADD, several testimonials, special offers, and multiple ways to purchase the product. And way below that, in tiny type, is the text: "The statements regarding these products have not been evaluated by the Food and Drug Administration. These products are not intended to diagnose, treat, cure or prevent any disease." What should you believe? The product is obviously named after "ADD," and the layout of the advertisement as well as their explicit claims tell you it treats all the symptoms of ADD. It boosts immune function, too! Many "supplement" advertisements clearly violate the intention of the FDA guidelines. Advertisements like this cannot be trusted.

The FTC and FDA allow certain health claims to be made by foods and supplements, including herbal products. (For more information about these regulations, visit www.cfsan.fda.gov/~dms/hclaims.html.) Some statements can include proven information about reducing the risk of diseases, though not treating or curing disease. For instance, products that contain the vitamin folic acid can say with FDA approval that "Folic acid may reduce the risk of certain birth defects." Other statements, known as "structure/function" claims, are not reviewed by the FDA and require no proof of their validity; rather, they're considered "dietary guidance." An example would be "Chondroitin promotes healthy bones." As long as the approved verbiage about not treating any disease is included, these kinds of statements are fair game and beyond the reach of regulatory authority. However, the content of these "structure/function" statements, which are supposed to only refer to maintaining normal structure or function, is often in practice stretched to make explicit health claims. An ADD supplement is said to "boost memory" and "increase attention," while Web sites trumpet chondriotin's ability to "stop crippling arthritis fast."

One reason the government pays much more attention to prescription and nonprescription advertising is because medications have more side effects, and are more likely to be harmful (see Chapter 10). But advertisements that make supplements and related products seem to be as dependable and useful as medications are deceptive. Be wary of all advertising, but especially wary of advertising for health products that evade the more stringent FDA regulations on medical products.

There are other sneaky ways to get around truth-in-advertising laws. Drug manufacturers can hire "paid endorsers." These can be health experts or celebrities paid to talk about how wonderful a product might be. Because it isn't the company making the claim, there's more leeway when an endorser speaks, and the endorser doesn't have to tell anyone that they've been paid to hawk the product. You'll hear a lot of these endorsements on AM radio. Avoid any "program" that sounds or looks suspiciously like an advertisement.

Product "informational campaigns" can lead to increased sales of a product without directly advertising anything. For instance, a very expensive product is available to help premature babies avoid serious respiratory infections. Though any direct advertising of the product would have to include all of the disclaimers and information about side effects, material mailed directly to parents informing them about these respiratory infections can skip of these important details as long as they don't directly mention the product. You're told about the disease, and are then encouraged to "talk to your doctor." This increases sales of the product, without any direct advertising at all. Similar informational campaigns led to a huge market for medicines treating "erectile dysfunction," a phrase that seemed to arise only after medicines could be sold to treat it. Informational campaigns themselves may provide good information, but they're just another form of advertising that has to be considered with suspicion.

The bottom line is that advertisements (including those that don't look like advertisements), should never be a primary source of information about

> ☞ **When looking for reliable health information, don't rely on advertising material. Even if it doesn't look like an ad, material that pays for placement or distribution cannot be trusted as a source of balanced information.**

health issues. Advertisers have their own motivations, and you can't expect them to look out for your interests.

An Insider's Guide to Suspicious Phrases

The same phrases appear over and over in misleading advertisements. Beware!

- "Scientific breakthrough!"
- "Ancient remedy!"
- "Secret ingredient!"
- "Revolutionary!"
- "Miracle!"

- "What the doctors won't tell you!"
- "NO drugs!"
- "100 percent safe! No side effects!"
- "Hurry!"
- "Really works!"
- "This is not a scam!"
- "Free trial!"
- "Money back guarantee!"

Extra punctuation and lots of capital letters are also a tip-off to an ad that's trying to rip you off. The most humorous claims combine these words into a real eye-opener: "This MIRACLE breakthrough product contains a revolutionary SECRET ingredient that really works!!! Hurry!!!!"

THE INTERNET AS A HEALTH INFORMATION RESOURCE

The Internet has become by far the most useful, and at times the most useless, source of information about everything, health included. Many well-meaning experts have written literally million of Web pages of information, and you can bet that if you've thought of a question chances are someone else has not only thought of it, but answered it. But how can parents best find the information they're looking for while avoiding the junk?

E-mail is one avenue for health information, but keep in mind that fraudulent e-mails are rampant. No one ensures the validity of e-mailed information. E-mails can live forever, circulating around and around as they're forwarded from one person to the next. Even information that was accurate when an e-mail was written can be irrelevant or misleading when it is read. Health care chain letters, in particular, should always be viewed with suspicion and deleted without following the ubiquitous instruction to "forward this to all of your friends." Be wary of information you receive in unsolicited e-mail, and refer to one of the trusted sites listed below to see if an e-mail's information is believable.

The World Wide Web is very much a public community; anyone with even minimal computer skills can write and publish whatever they want in a Web page. Though laws against slander and libel apply to material reproduced in Web pages, the sheer bulk of evolving Web material makes it very unlikely that anyone is vouching for the accuracy of most of the material on the Web.

These insider tips will let you know if a site is likely to be accurate and helpful:

- Web sites should make clear who is responsible for the site and its contents. There should be an "about us" type of link, including names, street addresses, and phone numbers. This information helps ensure that a genuine

organization, which presumably will have some fear of litigation should they promulgate misinformation, is behind the site.
- The authors and sources of information should be clear and well-referenced.
- Lookout for "references" that can't really be checked. "As seen on Oprah!" may look impressive, but there isn't enough information in the claim for anyone to check if it is true. A genuine reference includes exactly where you would need to look to confirm the information: "As reported in *Newsweek*, April 26, 1997."
- In general, the best health care Web sites are run by nonprofit organizations, government agencies, hospitals, universities, or private practitioners.
- Avoid commercial sites or sites that sell things.
- Be wary of product recommendations. Sites that sell the products they recommend are obviously suspect; but other sites that may seem to be unbiased may in fact receive "kick-backs" or other compensation by recommending certain medicines or other products. It may be difficult to know if such a relationship exists, but look to nonprofits, government, or other purely informational sites with clear ownership to be the most reliable. Collaborate recommendations from several sources rather than depend on any one site's recommendations.
- Avoid sites that seem biased or sectarian, representing a narrow point of view.
- Sites sponsored by drug companies or other commercial interests may indeed publish useful information, but should still be looked at with suspicion. It's better to depend on one of the many sites that do not have a sales-driven agenda.
- Sites run by support groups for specific individual diseases can be a mixed blessing. They may provide unique information about rare diseases, but may represent a narrow view of the disease that may or may not jibe with current science. Be wary of sites that seems unreasonable, or that don't clearly publish references for their material.
- Web sites should strive to stay current. Sites that do not put dates on articles may just be sloppy, or may be trying to deceive you.
- In general, informational sites should not try to collect any of your personal information. There should be no need to "register" or otherwise tell any site who you are or any other information about your family. If they're collecting this information, it is for marketing purposes. Move on to another site.
- Be careful about links to other sites. Some sites screen their links very carefully, and make this clear. Other sites will provide links to any other site for a fee. These should be marked as "sponsored links," but there is no requirement that this has to be done.
- Use common sense. Never depend on a single site as your only source of information, and keep in mind that if something sounds too good to be true, it probably is.

What Can You Learn about a Site from Its address?

If you look closely at a Web site's address, you can learn some useful hints. The string of characters after the http:// usually starts with a "www.", followed by a phrase that identifies the organization, followed by a period and then a short set of characters called the "top-level domain." There are only a few commonly seen top-level domains:

- .gov domains are only available to agencies of the United States government.
- .org domains are *traditionally* used by nonprofit organizations, but there is no requirement that any organization has to be nonprofit to use this designation. Anyone can purchase and use a .org domain.
- .com and .net domains can be used by anyone.
- .edu domains are restricted for use only by educational institutions. But students at these universities can set up their own Web sites using the .edu domain, potentially fooling someone into thinking that the university vouches for the content. These unregulated personal student sites will usually, but not always, look different from a genuine university site: their Web addresses will be longer and will often include a tilde (~) character.

Web Search Engines

Be careful. This evening I entered the phrase "children's health" into the most popular Web search site, retrieving 261 million results. The top three results listed are actually sites well-known to me with good information. But the fourth site listed turns out to be politically-oriented site, with hysterical and misguided information about imagined dangers in many ordinary household items. To a particularly gullible parent, this site would lead to anxiety and money down the drain—as the site prominently solicits for donations to fight for their cause.

You should also be aware of "sponsored sites," which pay to be displayed prominently in the search engines. That doesn't necessarily mean these sites are worthless, but you have to consider that they're paying extra money to get your attention. For the "children's health" search, the top sponsored sites were (1) an informational site about rotavirus, an important cause of diarrhea that just happens to be the target of a new vaccine; (2) a large soda manufacturer; and (3) a book publisher with some parenting and health books for sale. None of these "sponsored sites" were particularly useful for general-interest information about children's health, yet because of payments to the search site they're prominently featured. Skip the sponsored sites.

Useful and Dependable Sites

I've reviewed these sites for accuracy and usefulness, and to make sure that there are no conflicts of interest. There are very few commercial sites included, and any products that are sold are items well known and trusted by me. No pay sites are included. I have no commercial or ownership interest or any other relationship with the companies and individuals who run the sites listed in this book.

http://nccam.nih.gov/health/supplements.htm

Sponsored by the National Institutes of Health's Center for Complementary and Alternative Medicine, this site provides original articles as well as links to reputable articles from other sites about supplements that have undergone at least some scientific testing.

http://www.aap.org/

The official site of the AAP includes a parent's corner page with links to solid information about hundreds of health topics. The front page usually has links to in-depth information about whatever's currently in the news about children's health. This site does include a store from which AAP-sponsored publications can be published, including many excellent books for parents on health and behavior topics.

http://www.ahrq.gov/

Sponsored by the Agency for Healthcare Research and Quality, part of the United States Department of Health and Human Services, this site's best information is about choosing and using health insurance plans. Look under the "Consumers" link for information on "Health Plans." The site also includes good information about preventing medical errors, communicating clearly with your doctor, and using prescription medications safely.

http://www.bemboszoo.com/

Just for fun, a cool and mesmerizing site. Your kids will enjoy it too.

http://www.cdc.gov/

This is a huge but well-organized Web site sponsored by the United States Government's Centers for Disease Control. Among the most useful sections are areas about traveler's health, environmental health, and the opening page's links to current health news topics.

http://www.cfsan.fda.gov/

The FDA's Center for Food Safety and Applied Nutrition works to ensure that foods and cosmetics are safe and honestly labeled. Its Web site includes excellent, unbiased, and in-depth articles about many subjects, including regulatory issues, food additives, pesticide contaminants, bioterrorism, food allergens, and infant formula.

http://www.childrensnyp.org/

Two children's hospitals sponsor this site, which includes a truly encyclopedic list of articles concerning just about any children's health problem. Click on "Child health A to Z" for the list.

http://www.eatright.org

Click on the link to "Food and Nutrition Information" for some well-researched and useful information about diet and nutrition from the American Dietetic Association.

http://www.fda.gov/

The United States FDA's homepage has extensive links to regulatory and other information about the safe use of medicines and medical devices.

http://www.ftc.gov/bcp/conline/edcams/cureall/

An excellent site run by the United States Federal Trade Commission, "Operation Cure.All" is a program designed to identify false or misleading Internet health claims through enforcement of truth-in-advertising laws and consumer education. There are links to about a dozen specific articles designed to help consumers spot fraudulent sites, as well as links to other government and private sector sites with solid, reliable health information.

http://www.healthfinder.gov/

Run by the United States Department of Health and Human Services, this is a somewhat overwhelming site that attempts to organize and link to a great number of prescreened health sites on the Web. Federal, state, nonprofit, and professional organizations are all accessible through this site, which claims to have reviewed each represented organization to ensure reliable information.

http://www.insurekidsnow.gov/

The United States Department of Health and Human Services runs this site, designed to help families arrange for free or low-cost health insurance plans. Every state has its own health care plans in place for children from low-income families, and links from this central site can get you started. You'll also find good general information about low-cost insurance and immigration issues.

http://www.keepkidshealthy.com/

Run by a pediatrician, this is an extensive site with lots of "first-hand" information. There are online tools including a height predictor, body-mass index calculator, and baby name generator; there's also a very useful and searchable list of product recalls. A link to an "ask the pediatrician" forum leads to some useful advice and give-and-take by parents, but when I reviewed it the forum didn't seem to include too many posts from an actual pediatrician.

http://www.kidshealth.org/

Featuring subsites for parents, kids, and teens, KidsHealth is run by the nonprofit Nemours Foundation. Superb and interesting articles about parenting and health issues are found at the parents' site, while children of all ages can safely find responsible and age-appropriate information about health at their own sections. Teenagers in particular can rely on this site for honest and reliable information that they may not get in other places.

http://www.nlm.nih.gov/medlineplus/childrenshealth.html

This site features summaries of recently-published scientific articles about children's health, along with links to many general-interest children's health resources. If you read a summary of a new study in the newspaper and want to find out more information, this is a good place to start.

http://www.parenting.org/

Girls and Boys Town is a nonprofit organization that helps care for troubled and difficult children. Their site includes information about ordinary parenting issues that arise for children at every age, as well as information about how to contact them for a referral to local services or agencies for parents who find themselves in a crisis.

http://www.quackwatch.org/

Run by a retired psychiatrist, this is an eye-opening site that coldly and rationally reports on health care fraud and abuse. All of the articles are extensively referenced. There's an extensive list of just about every kind of alternative health care system and product, linking to articles that elaborate on their claims and any scientific evidence for or against their effectiveness. There's also extensive information for consumers on how to critically evaluate health care products and theories, with a goal of saving you money and harm. If you've heard overly-glowing claims about any sort of "fringe" health care item, check out this site for "the rest of the story" *before* you spend your money.

http://www.thesafeside.com/

It can be difficult to talk to children about the dangers posed by strangers—you want your children to be safe and alert, but you don't want them too fearful to play outside. This superb site offers guidance for teachers and parents about how to help kids learn to be safe outside. The site also sells an entertaining video for children age five to ten about staying safe with strangers.

http://www.vaccineinformation.org/

To me, this is the single best source for accurate and up-to-date information about vaccines and vaccine-preventable diseases. Its sister site, www.immunize.org, is more geared to health professionals but nonetheless has very useful information for parents as well. Both are run by the nonprofit Immunization Action Coalition, and all information is scrupulously reviewed by their large list of expert consultants. These are not just rah-rah vaccine sites; they do clearly run through the shortcomings and adverse reactions that are possible with vaccines, while doing an excellent job of illustrating the importance of continued vaccination as a key public health measure.

http://www.wikipedia.org/

This is a fascinating site. Think of it as the biggest encyclopedia you've ever encountered, with over a million articles in English on just about any topic, including health issues. The articles are written by anyone who wishes to contribute, and can further be edited by anyone else with an interest in the subject. You can find some excellent information about even the most obscure health issues here, including links to other Web sources; but keep in mind that the articles are certainly not guaranteed to be accurate. Still, the Wikipedia community does a remarkably good job of identifying and fixing erroneous information.

http://www.williamgladdenfoundation.org/

This nonprofit organization provides free access to hundreds of articles about behavioral, discipline, and mental health issues affecting children and families. Though there are sponsored links along the left and right sides, these are clearly identified and won't interfere with your taking advantage of the great amount of excellent information available through this site.

13

REVEALED: THE MAGIC
OF LABS AND TESTS

Blood tests, urine tests, x-rays, ultrasounds, EKGs—the number of high technology tests a doctor can order is staggering and mystifying. And these kinds of tests are magical, too. They can reveal exactly what's going on inside of your child, right?

Wrong.

Why do patients love tests? Perhaps they really can give you an exact, accurate answer. They're formal and ritualized, and often give you numbers that can be quoted, compared, and looked up on the Internet. They can be ranked, and categorized, and printed neatly by a machine. A test is cold, authoritative, and correct.

Why to physicians love tests? We get numbers, and ranges of exactly what's "normal." They allow us to lean on someone else's judgment, and give us extra certainty and wisdom. A test, unlike a subjective physical exam, won't let you down.

Wrong, wrong, wrong.

It turns out that tests are as fallible and prone to errors as people, sometimes more so. They're ordered for the wrong reasons and can mislead both the doctor and patient, distracting from what really might be the problem. They're expensive, too, and for kids many of them can be painful and frightening. Many tests done at a radiology department expose children to ionizing radiation, which will slightly increase their lifetime risk of cancer.

But don't misunderstand: there certainly are times when tests and procedures can be critically important to help your pediatrician make a diagnosis or plan of care. Being able to do a simple, reliable swab to confirm strep throat ensures that antibiotics aren't used unnecessarily; a CT scan can quickly determine if a child needs immediate surgery after a serious car wreck. The right test can be lifesaving.

In this chapter we'll look at tests: what they can do, and what they cannot do. There are many kinds of tests in medicine: laboratory tests on blood or urine or other fluids; radiology exams with x-rays, ultrasounds, radioactive particles, or magnets and radio waves; electrocardiograms (EKGs, also sometimes abbreviated "ECGs") and electroencephalograms (EEGs); stress tests; biopsies; even psychologic tests based on panels of questions. All of these tests share common characteristic shortcomings and problems that you ought to know about before they're performed on our child.

All Tests Are "Inaccurate" to Some Degree

Some tests are better than others, but any test can be misleading or inaccurate. There are many different ways a test can go wrong.

- *The sample was collected on the wrong patient, or mislabeled.* Unfortunately, this is common. Be especially wary if your child has a common name, or if you know there is another child with the same name in your pediatrician's practice.
- *The test was performed incorrectly.* Tests need to be performed exactly the right way. Even simple office based tests can have pitfalls. For instance, a home pregnancy test read a few minutes too late may become falsely positive; if read too early, it may show as negative. Tests performed infrequently are less likely to be done correctly.
- *The test was interpreted incorrectly.* Labs often have "reference ranges" of normal values. The posted ranges may not be correct in pediatric patients because normal results vary according to the age of the child. Some tests, such as EKGs, require considerable expertise to interpret correctly.
- *Some drug or other substance interfered with the test.* Antihistamines can make allergy skin testing invalid; eating prior to a measurement of cholesterol can change the results. Before an endoscopy procedure, steps need to be taken to clean out the bowel. If a child isn't correctly prepared for the test, you may not be able to rely on the results.
- *The doctor didn't understand what the results of the tests mean, and reported them incorrectly.* You would hope that before physicians order tests they know exactly what to expect from the results, and will know exactly what the results mean. If something truly unusual comes up, physicians need to discuss it with a knowledgeable colleague before unnecessarily worrying the family. If you get the impression that your physician is not confident about what the results of a test mean, ask for a referral to an appropriate specialist.
- *Tests are meant to uncover specific problems; there is no such thing as a test that will tell you "everything."* A patient might tell me, "I was tested by the allergist and I'm not allergic to anything." Apart from the fact that allergy tests themselves are not always accurate, no one can possibly be tested for allergy to anything and everything. What an allergist can test is for allergies to common things, or things that appear to be likely from a patient's history. If those tests are negative, the correct interpretation from the allergist ought to be "It is unlikely that you are allergic to the things I tested you for."
- *An incorrect test may occur for a predictable medical reason.* For instance, a chest x-ray can be performed to evaluate a child for pneumonia. It detects areas of increased density in the chest indicating the presence of excess fluid that

may be infected. But if your child is dehydrated from fever and vomiting, a chest x-ray can be normal at first. After the child keeps down some fluids, a repeated x-ray may well show that pneumonia. A good clinician knows the limits of the tests, and when the results can't be trusted.

• *Sometimes, even when everything is done and interpreted correctly, a test can still be inaccurate.* Nothing is perfect. If the test result really doesn't fit the situation, repeat it or ignore it. Better yet, physicians should not perform a test if they already know they won't believe an abnormal result.

Two kinds of results are incorrect:

• A *"False positive"* test tells you that something is wrong when in fact it is not.
• A *"False negative"* test tells you that everything is OK, when in fact a problem is present.

Either can be a problem, depending on the situation. Some tests are designed to minimize false negative results, especially tests used to screen for common conditions (for example, a newborn hearing screen). Other tests by design have very few false positives, like a test confirming an HIV infection. In general, you can't have it both

> ☞ **No test is perfect.**

ways—most single tests are designed to minimize either the false negatives or false positives. Your clinician needs to understand this to choose and interpret tests correctly for your particular circumstances.

IF YOU DO ENOUGH TESTS, ONE WILL BE WRONG

Let's say that a certain blood test is 95 percent accurate, that is, you'll get an incorrect result only 5 percent of the time, or one in twenty times the test is run. That's pretty good odds, right?

The problem is that many tests are done in panels, or groups of tests. A common blood panel may comprise twenty individual tests. What if each of these has 95 percent accuracy? Now, since you're actually doing twenty tests, there's a very good chance that at least one of these will yield an incorrect result. In fact, if you perform twenty tests, each of which is incorrect 5 percent of the time, more than half of the time *at least one* of the tests in the panel will be incorrect.

To help illustrate this, think about drawing a card from a deck that includes jokers. If you pull a joker, that would be like getting an inaccurate result on a test. With a desk of fifty-two cards and two jokers, you have about a 4 percent chance of pulling a joker if you draw one card from one deck. But what if you have to draw a card from each of ten or twenty decks? As you can imagine, the more decks of cards you draw

> ☞ **The more tests you do, the more misinformation you'll get.**

from the higher a chance that at least once you'll get that joker. In other words, the more tests you do, the more the chance that one will we abnormal, even if nothing is wrong.

For those of you who want more details, the mathematical background for examples like these are in the appendix.

IF THE DISEASE IS VERY UNLIKELY, A POSITIVE TEST RESULT IS PROBABLY WRONG

Again, if you wish to become an "advanced insider," the mathematical details for this section are in the appendix. But even without going into the math, let me provide some examples to help you understand another important limitation of tests.

Let's use our chest x-ray example again. This test is quite accurate; for the sake of this example we'll say 96 percent of people with pneumonia will have an abnormal chest x-ray. So what does this mean, if *your* child has an abnormal chest x-ray? Here's two scenarios that illustrate how important it is to consider how likely it is the child has pneumonia *before* the chest x-ray is performed:

1. Aunt Marge has pneumonia, and your son has a cough. He has no fever, and isn't particularly ill. You tell the doctor, "I know he really isn't acting sick, and I know he probably doesn't have pneumonia, but can you do a chest x-ray to make sure?" In this case, with no symptoms of pneumonia except cough, the chance that your child really has pneumonia is very low, let's say 4–5 percent. Even if his x-ray is abnormal his chance of *really* having pneumonia is only about 50 percent. You might have just flipped a coin; that would give you the same insight as the chest x-ray without the radiation and expense!
2. Your child has a fever of 103.6, a cough, and is breathing rapidly. With this presentation, his likelihood of having pneumonia is fairly high, let's say 30 percent. In this circumstance an abnormal chest x-ray would predict that his chance of truly having pneumonia would be 90 percent.

In all circumstances, if the chances of a child actually having a disease are very low, even a test that is very accurate will have a high number of false results. Because many tests have low accuracy, they should only be performed in circumstances where the likelihood of truly having disease is high. Otherwise, tests are far more likely to mislead than to be helpful.

Let's go through one more example, using a different sort of test. Many states now mandate that all newborns undergo a hearing exam. Hearing problems in newborns are fairly common (about six newborns out of every thousand have a significant hearing problem), and early identification and treatment can allow these kids to lead more ordinary lives. In this case, a screening test is applied to children who have a low probability of disease, just to catch the few who really have hearing loss. Using the most common screening tool, if your child "fails" his newborn screening exam, the chance that he really has a problem is about one in ten. That is, for every ten kids who fail the screening test, nine will be perfectly normal when retested with more elaborate equipment. This doesn't mean it is a bad test or a bad idea, but this explanation needs to be available to every worried parent whose kid fails the screen!

As More Tests Are Performed the Level of Anxiety Increases, Whatever the Tests' Results

This has more to do with human nature than the nature of tests, but in my experience this statement is absolutely true.

> Eight-year-old P.J. comes in complaining of belly pain. By the history, it is clear that most of his belly pain is occurring on school days. This may be because school itself is stressful, or it may be that he tends to skip breakfast those days. A reasonable course of action would be to discuss this with the family, have the child eat breakfast every day, and keep a diary of symptoms to really get a handle on what's going on. Follow-up is suggested in two weeks to review progress.

Instead, let's say that this particular pediatrician says "Well, this seems to be a school day problem, but let's run some tests to make absolutely sure." Now, you already know that statement doesn't really make sense—no tests are ever so accurate to be "absolutely sure"—but the family goes ahead with the plan for several blood and stool tests. If they're all normal, the family and child are still anxious. They wonder if

☞ **If the diagnosis is clear, no tests are necessary. Unneeded tests increase worry and anxiety.**

the right tests were done, or they wonder if something serious was missed. Even worse: if one of the tests comes back abnormal, even if it's obviously an incorrect result the family will be very anxious and will end up going through more tests!

Tests Should Be Done to Confirm a Diagnosis, Not to "Fish" for a Diagnosis

Doctors are not infallible, and patients do not always have the "typical" or obvious symptoms explained in textbooks. Many times a diagnosis is suspected but not confirmed after the physicians' history and physical exam. This is when a test is the most valuable.

But sometimes a physician, or the patient themselves, asks for tests "just to see if something is wrong." As we've been discussing, this is very unlikely to yield any useful information. In fact, if a test done in this manner is abnormal, it is more likely to be wrong (a "false positive") than correct. Most tests are just not accurate enough to be used for mass screenings in people who are very unlikely to have a truly abnormal result. In other words, unexpected results are seldom helpful.

One good example of this is mass screenings of high-school students for heart problems using an echocardiogram to prevent sudden unexpected death in athletes. Unfortunately, even with the best equipment and technicians, far more "false positives" are discovered than are children really at risk for dying. In other words, most of the kids who have an abnormal result on this kind of screening are in fact perfectly fine with no increased risk of death. After testing of this sort, many families will be needlessly anxious. Even worse, no one has ever shown that doing these sorts of screenings prevents deaths. Even in the best of circumstances, an echocardiogram can only diagnose a minority of the conditions that can predispose to sudden death. A normal screening echocardiogram does not eliminate the risk of dying on the playing field. A far more effective strategy that would certainly save more lives would be to use the money for dietary, exercise, and other healthy lifestyle counseling and activities.

SOME TESTS MIGHT REVEAL INFORMATION THAT YOU DON'T WANT TO KNOW

Mom decided to have her four sons' blood types tested, because she read somewhere on the Internet that blood types can help predict future personality issues. It turns out that one child has blood type B positive. Her own blood type is O negative, and her husband's blood type is A positive. The parents brought these results to me for interpretation.

Put yourself in the pediatrician's shoes. Would you tell this nice family, with a stable marriage and a father who thinks he's the biologic parent of four boys that his paternity is in doubt?

Other examples of this sort of "you just don't want to know" result might include results that show a child has an increased risk of a disease that won't begin until they're an adult. In this case, do you want to know? Do you want your child to know? How about a future employer or a future health insurance company? Think through what the results of a test might mean to your family and your child *before* you perform the test.

SOME TESTS ENTAIL RISKS FROM ANESTHESIA OR RADIATION

To perform some tests, including biopsies and lengthy radiology procedures like MRI scans, your child will have to be sedated. Though the risk is very small, there is a chance of a serious or deadly reaction to anesthetic agents. If you have a young child, you should ensure that anesthesia is only administered by practitioners with pediatric training and expertise, in a setting where any adverse event can quickly be addressed.

Radiation exposure is another small but real risk posed by some tests. By one estimate 0.5 percent of cancers—that is, 5 out of 1000—are a direct result of diagnostic radiology procedures. Radiation exposure to children (who have far more years to live than adults) is more likely to lead to an eventual cancer years later. Many physicians do not seriously consider the risk of the radiation exposure when they are ordering tests on their patients. The most radiation exposure comes from CT scans and fluoroscopy, followed by ordinary x-rays. Nuclear medicine procedures like bone scans expose the patient to very little radiation. Ultrasounds and MRI scans carry no risk from radiation exposure.

To keep radiation risks in perspective: remember that all of us, all of the time, are constantly bombarded with radiation from natural and unavoidable sources. So there is no way to eliminate our risks. A simple chest x-ray adds radiation exposure equivalent to what you would have gotten in about 2.5 days of natural background exposure—that's not too much extra. But a typical barium enema study is equivalent to an extra 2.3 years of exposure, and a typical abdominal CT scan can expose your child to the equivalent of an extra 3.3 years of natural radiation exposure. I'm certainly not suggesting that these studies should never be done, but their need must be weighed against their risks.

Some tips can help minimize your child's risks from diagnostic radiology procedures:

- The younger the child, the more important it is to minimize radiation exposures.
- Avoid repeated studies and procedures when possible.
- Use lead or bismuth shielding over body parts that don't need to be imaged; only the body part in question needs to be exposed.
- If appropriate, an MRI or ultrasound study eliminates any radiation risk and may be a reasonable substitute for a CT scan.
- Rely on imaging centers that perform many studies on children and have made the best effort to use the smallest dose of radiation possible. Radiology departments that see children infrequently are more likely to use more radiation, and more likely to have to repeat a botched study.
- Try to get a good image the first time. Help your child settle down and get into position. A poorly done study is worse than no study at all, and repeating films means more and more exposures.
- Body parts that are probably the most sensitive to radiation include the gonads, thyroid gland (in the front of the neck), and girl's chests. Keep these parts shielded or avoid imaging them entirely if possible.
- Have copies made of radiology studies to bring to specialists so they don't need to be repeated.
- Some centers have ultrafast CT scanners that use much less radiation and take much less time—that means anesthesia may not be needed. They're not

available in all communities, but try to have your child's study done with one of these newer scanners if possible.
- Most importantly, perform these and all other tests only if they're clinically necessary.

Should a Test Be Done?

To summarize, there are some valid reasons why a test should *not* be performed:

- They hurt.
- They're expensive.
- They can mislead with an abnormal result that's wrong.
- They can mislead with a normal result that's wrong.
- They can increase anxiety.
- They may have unintended consequences.
- Some tests expose your child to risks from radiation or anesthesia.

On the other hand, tests can sometimes be an essential tool to help make medical decisions.

- Tests can help decide a treatment plan, especially when there are different ways to treat possible diagnoses.
- Tests can help zero in on a diagnosis when there are many possible explanations for a child's symptoms.
- Tests can reliably exclude a very serious diagnosis that cannot be "ruled out" even after a thorough history and physical exam.

Don't Assume No News Is Good News

Don't assume that the results are normal if you haven't heard from your doctor. Expect the office to contact you with all results, normal or abnormal; if you haven't heard from them in a reasonable time, pick up the phone.

Labs and tests are certainly very useful to confirm a suspected diagnosis, or rule out a possible diagnosis that is especially serious. But as we've seen they can be very misleading, especially if they are ordered for the wrong reasons. With your insider's knowledge, you should be able to better understand what labs and tests can and cannot tell you about your child's health.

14

CHOOSING INSURANCE AND PAYING BILLS: HOW TO SPEND LESS AND GET MORE

Medical care is expensive. If your employer offers medical insurance as a benefit, take it. In many cases, you'll have no choice between plans; just take whatever's offered. But for those of you who work for larger companies that offer a choice of plans, or for those who have to make their own arrangements for health insurance, be prepared with the best insider tips to help you with your choice. Choosing the right insurance plan can protect you from the exclusion of preexisting conditions, can prevent you from having high out-of-pocket costs, and can allow you freedom to choose your own physicians and health care facilities. However, insurance plans that are the friendliest for patients are often the most expensive. To make the best choice, you'll need to balance the benefits of better plans against their higher costs.

Whether or not you were able to choose your health insurance plan, families can still end up spending a bundle on health care services. Insurance companies will try their best to avoid paying the bills, hoping that at least some of their customers give up and pay the bills themselves. Your insurance carrier can legitimately refuse to pay some items if those are excluded in your contract, but there is a lot of wiggle room where persistence and insider knowledge can help you get more for your money.

HEALTH CARE PLANS

When choosing health insurance, the first decision to make is whether to participate in a group plan (often offered through an employer) or to buy an individual plan. In almost all cases, it is best to be part of a group plan because of its unique advantages:

- Premiums are cheaper.
- When paid by or through an employer, group plans can be purchased with pretax dollars—in effect further reducing their cost to you.
- You are better protected against the exclusion of "preexisting medical conditions."

There are some advantages of an individual plan:

- They may be the only choice available if there is no employer who will purchase group insurance for you.
- If you do buy your own individual plan, you can pick exactly the plan you want.

Preexisting medical conditions may be excluded from coverage when you apply for health insurance. A new insurance company can refuse to pay for the care of those conditions and complications of those conditions. Fortunately, the picture is not so dire: by federal law (called HIPAA), if you are covered under a group plan and switch to a different group plan, the second plan *cannot* exclude any preexisting health conditions. However, if you are uninsured or a member of an individual plan, a newly joined group plan can exclude any preexisting conditions from coverage for up to one year.

For most families, the advantages of an employer-purchased group plan outweigh those of an individual plan. Even if you are self-employed or your employer does not offer coverage, you may be able to purchase group heath insurance through a civic association, professional club, or religious organization.

If you must purchase your own individual plan, look for a "noncancelable" or "guaranteed renewable" policy. If you've purchased this and pay your premiums on time, the insurance company can't drop your coverage. They might be able to cancel their entire insurance line for everyone, but they can't drop you individually even if you run up high costs.

For most group plans, once you've made your choice you cannot change until the next "open enrollment" period. These typically occur only once a year.

Many families do not get a choice of plan. The employer offers one insurance policy, and employees can take it or leave it (at least until the employer changes plans). If you are given only one option for employer-sponsored health insurance, take it. For those working for larger companies, or those who have to choose their own plan, there are some varieties to consider.

Traditional (Also Called "Indemnity" or "Fee for Service")

This is the old-fashioned health insurance your parents had. They went to any doctor or used any medical facility, and the insurance company paid most of their bills after a modest deductible. That's what's supposed to happen—but it turns out that even this premium and expensive insurance has sneaky tricks that can leave families stuck with huge medical bills.

After you've met the deductible, most indemnity plans pay 80 percent of what's called the "usual and customary charge" for services. The 20 percent that you have to pay is called the "coinsurance." If your physician charged more than the usual and customary amount, you have to pay both the "coinsurance" and whatever amount is above that usual and customary figure. This can lead to enormous medical bills because each insurance company determines their own usual and customary figure. This may be well below what is actually charged.

Johnny is two years old, and has always been in good health. One night he develops a fever and cough. At the local emergency room, he is evaluated by a physician and receives blood tests, a chest x-ray, and intravenous antibiotics. The bills for the hospital services total up like this:

	Charge
ER visit	$450
Supplies	$160
ER physician's fee	$150
X-ray	$200
Radiologist's fee	$120
Lab fees	$110
Total	$1190

However, the "Explanation of Benefits" from the insurance company looks like this:

	Charge	"Usual and Customary Fee"
ER visit	$450	$110
Supplies	$160	$35
ER physician's fee	$150	$145
X-ray	$200	$60
Radiologist's fee	$120	$110
Lab fees	$110	$55
Total	$1190	$515

The insurance company will pay only 80 percent of their usual and customary, or $412. Of course, you have a $250 deductible as well— so for a bill of $1,190, the insurance will pay $162, and you're stuck with a bill for $1,028. This scenario is not uncommon with indemnity insurance.

The insurance company's estimates of usual and customary charges can be appealed, but many families don't bother with the hassle—which is exactly what the insurers are counting on to cut their costs. There are no regulations that spell out exactly what is considered usual and customary, and insurers will typically not share these figures with you until after the procedure is done and billed. Later in this chapter, we'll go over the best ways to appeal an insurance company's payment decisions, including unreasonable benefit reductions for underestimated "usual and customary" charges.

Fee-for-service insurance is available, but expensive. And using it is a hassle: you have to keep very careful records, file your own claims, and be prepared to fight if bills aren't paid. Though sick care and prescriptions are typically covered, health maintenance visits (check-ups) are not. For most people, indemnity insurance is no longer the best option. One of the managed care schemes, either a Preferred Provider Organization (PPO) or Health Maintenance Organization (HMO), will usually provide good health care access with more predictable and controllable costs.

Preferred Provider Organization (PPO)

Though their premiums are less costly than those of traditional insurance, PPOs are still expensive. You can visit any of the doctors in a provider directory, and usually almost any hospital, imaging center, or laboratory is a participant. No referral is needed from a primary physician for specialty care. Compared with HMOs, PPOs don't have tight restrictions on who you can see and how you can see them. There is usually a substantial copay for each visit, but the convenience of going to a broad number of places without worrying about referrals may be worth the extra cost. Often, PPO plans exclude or limit certain kinds of health care, which may mean no coverage for well child visits or immunizations. (Your county health department can administer the same immunizations as your pediatrician at a lower cost. If your insurance doesn't cover immunizations, go to your county health department and bring the records to your pediatrician.)

Other kinds of care that might be specifically excluded include mental health issues (including school problems or attention deficit disorder), speech problems, or developmental disorders. Many people with PPO-based insurance have a high deductible that must be reached before the PPO covers anything. There is usually some provision for out-of-network benefits at a substantial penalty. If you go out of network, you'll typically have to pay an extra deductible plus coinsurance, which can include costs for charges that exceed the "usual and customary" amounts—basically meaning you have to pay for anything the insurance company doesn't want to pay! But again, in most PPOs the provider list is extensive, and most people would not need to go outside of the PPO network.

> ☞ **For PPOs and HMOs, the single best way to control your costs is to stay in the plan's network.**

Health Maintenance Organization (HMO)

This variety of insurance is favored by many employers because premiums are the least expensive. Participants choose from a fairly limited number of "primary providers" who will act as their main contact for health concerns. For children, the primary physicians are usually pediatricians. Visits to the doctor usually cost only a small copay. For ordinary well child care HMO coverage is excellent. It typically includes all recommended vaccines, well child visits, and usual tests and procedures done as part of routine well care. The problem with HMO coverage begins when a child is actually ill. In order to

> ☞ **For any health care services, an HMO will only cover the bill if the service provider is part of the HMO directory *and* the primary physician has obtained permission for the service from the HMO (a so-called "referral"). If the service provider is not in network, or no referral has been done, *you* will be responsible for the entire bill.**

see any specialist, the primary physician must be seen first to obtain a referral. Failure to get a proper referral could mean that specialist visits will not be covered, even if the specialist is in the network. Because HMO networks tend to include smaller numbers of physicians, expect some waits to get in to see a specialist. Also, keep in mind that not only is physician access restricted, but so is your choice of lab or radiology facilities. Just because an assigned primary physician sent a patient to a certain imaging center for an x-ray doesn't mean that the imaging center or its radiologists participate in the HMO network. And that leaves the patient responsible for the bill.

With an HMO, personally call your HMO to make sure that they will cover a specialty, radiology, or lab visit *before* the visit takes place. Though most of us who provide care to HMO patients try to avoid antagonizing parents by sending people to the wrong places, the myriad of changing rules of each HMO means that mistakes will happen.

For emergency or after-hours care, HMO members can usually go to any emergency department. Check with the HMO directly about care through urgent care centers. Always call your primary physician's office the next business day after an ER visit to make sure that they request the referral. Though many Emergency Departments will fax a referral request to the primary physician, you can't depend on this. It's your money!

Some HMOs, called "group models," employ their own doctors and set up their own separate facilities where you must go to seek care. This can be simpler for the patients—anything in the HMO building is always covered, including radiology services, tests, and pharmacy—but if you're enrolled in this kind of plan you must visit this central clinic for all of your health care needs.

Point of Service (POS)

This is a hybrid plan, based on a somewhat liberalized HMO model. You can see specialists within the plan without a referral from your primary physician, and there is at least some coverage for services by providers outside the network. POS plans vary widely in their rules and set-up, so you'll have to look closely at the rules for a particular plan to decide if a POS is worth the higher premiums compared to a traditional HMO.

Does Your Pediatrician Care What Insurance You Have?

The answer should be "no." Good practices strive to treat all of their patients identically, as much as possible. In some cases, tests or labs done by your pediatrician will only be reimbursed by certain plans, so some families will be referred to outside facilities for these items. Offices also have to keep track of your plan's details to know if referrals are needed, or what community resources are "in-network" for you. These strategies are used by conscientious practices to help minimize your out-of-pocket expenses.

This has been a general overview of the most common types of health insurance coverage. Keep in mind that the exact plan you've been offered may not exactly follow the rules above. When evaluating any health plan, look into the specific details offered by your employer or insurance representative.

PLAN BENEFITS

Not all health care plans cover all of the benefits you might expect. For instance, indemnity insurance and PPOs are less likely to cover preventive health services. Look at this list of health benefits and see if a plan you're considering covers the items that are most important to you:

- Check-ups and health screening items
- Routine immunizations
- Hospital and emergency care
- Services at "urgent care centers"
- Vision
- Dental
- Prescription medications
- Mental health
- Rehabilitative care including speech therapy, physical therapy, and occupational therapy
- Alternative care such as chiropractic

You may not know which of these will be the most important to you in the future, but be especially aware of big-ticket items such as hospital and emergency services. If your child has chronic health issues requiring ongoing care, be sure to find out if these items will be covered.

Find out if a plan you are considering has a cap on out-of-pocket expenses per year for each family—this works to your advantage if a disaster strikes. On the other hand, some plans will cap their own "lifetime expenses," so that no matter what happens, they will only pay a total of a million dollars, lifetime, for any of your children's care. Though of course the chance that a child will need more than this is slim, one million dollars may not last as long as you think if a truly terrible and chronic health problem strikes. Be aware of this potential limitation written into some insurance contracts.

READ THE CONTRACT

An insurance contract can be difficult to read thoroughly and carefully. You probably won't get a copy until after you've signed up; you may not get a copy at all if you don't ask for it. To further confound you, the contract is probably written in barely comprehensible legalese. Still, pour yourself some coffee and read through the contract so you know exactly what expenses are going to be covered. Keep these insider tips in mind while reviewing a health insurance contract:

- Benefit exclusions can be hidden in the fine print.
- Don't assume that your employer knows exactly how a plan works. Health plans are often purchased through brokers who themselves may not have studied the contracts, and many employers go straight to the price rather than get caught up in the details of exactly what is covered.
- Be especially aware of the distinction between "emergency" and "urgent" care. These can end up being a tremendous out-of-pocket cost. Any health insurance should cover care that is needed in an emergency, but some plans will be more picky about exactly what "emergency" means. Find out in advance what steps are necessary to ensure emergency care coverage, rather than have to fight through a phone tree while your child is sick.
- Be especially wary when reading about the coverage requirements for referrals, preexisting conditions, covered versus non-covered services, and emergency care. Study the sections called "exclusions and limitations" to avoid unpleasant surprises.

IF YOU'VE LOST YOUR INSURANCE

For many families, a loss of employment means that insurance coverage is terminated. Federal law can help in this situation. Referred to as "COBRA" coverage, employers who have health insurance benefits and more than twenty employees must offer continued group health insurance coverage for employees who lose their job. Employees are eligible for COBRA coverage whether they quit, were fired, or laid off—as long as they have not committed "gross misconduct." You can also qualify for COBRA coverage in cases of divorce or the death of an insured spouse. You'll have to pay the premium yourself—which can be more expensive than the discounted premium your employer paid—and you have a limited time after leaving the job to elect to get this coverage. Still, it's better than no coverage at all while you're looking for a new job. Staying on a COBRA plan will also prevent the next group insurance carrier from excluding any preexisting conditions.

Blood from a Stone

We've talked about the biggest chunk of health care costs and how they are paid, including doctor visits, hospitals, labs, and radiology services. But there are other costs that can become significant, including prescription drugs, mental health, and rehabilitative services. Insurance companies try to aggressively avoid payments for these items, even more so than for more ordinary medical expenses. There are of course insider tricks to minimizing your own costs for these items your insurance company doesn't cover.

Keep in mind that the insurance company will make the final decision on payment. But that does not mean that the insurance company has made the final decision on whether or not your child can get the services. There are times where you will need to spend your own money on a needed medicine, or speech therapy, or visits to a psychiatrist. Or you may be in an urgent situation where you must commit to paying for services yourself, even while working with the insurance company to see if coverage is available. If you're in this situation, make sure the medical provider knows you're a "self-paying" patient; there may be discounts. Also, try to spend this sort of money out of a health care savings account or flexible health care spending account.

Prescription Drugs

Many health insurance plans include prescription drug benefits. These can be very valuable especially if used to their full advantage. Most plans have a list of covered drugs; some divide medications into two or more tiers of increasing copays. Though the plans will send booklets of covered prescription products to their doctors, most of us who see patients from a variety of plans cannot keep up with these ever-changing lists. Beyond trying to pick drugs from the least expensive categories, there are other tricks to minimize your out of pocket expenses for prescriptions.

- Ask your doctor to prescribe medicines that are available in generic form. There are usually plenty of generic choices for a particular use, and generics are every bit as good as branded products. Newer, pricier drugs are promoted very heavily for physicians to prescribe. But older generics are often just as effective and safer than brand name products. Generic products will always be available at the lowest copay.

- If the pharmacist tells you a medicine is not covered or requires a high copay, ask if there are alternatives. You can also call your prescription benefit company for suggested "therapeutic substitutes." You or the pharmacist can call your doctor to request a change.
- Ask your pediatrician for samples. These are often available for newer brand name medicines.
- For medicines that are needed long term, many insurance plans have a "mail in" scheme for medications. You can get a three months supply at a reduced copay if you mail in your prescription. This will be cheaper than purchasing your medicine month to month at a local pharmacy.
- It may be possible for your physician to prescribe a larger quantity of an expensive drug, so you get more for the same copay. This can be especially useful for prescription skin products or for medicines that are taken "as needed." Note that the pharmacy is usually limited to dispensing a thirty day supply, so a doctor's prescription for more than thirty pills of a once-a-day medicine will be filled for only thirty days. But for products that are measured less exactly than pills, larger quantities than a typical month's supply can be filled for one copay.
- Some pills can be split, allowing you to get "two for the price of one." For example, if your child needs 100 mg of "Gentlemycin" a day for long term control of acne, your pediatrician might be able to prescribe 200 mg tablets that you can then cut in half with a pill cutter. This won't work for every medicine—time release pills and capsules can't be split. If your child is on a long-term expensive medication, ask your doctor if pill splitting can save you money.
- Medicines can sometimes be purchased at a lower cost from outside the United States, usually from Canada. As this scheme has become more popular, many illegitimate businesses have gotten into the act, so ask for first hand recommendations rather than rely on Internet pop-up ads to find a reliable and honest Canadian pharmacy.
- Many drug manufacturers offer free or reduced price medicines through their own "Patient Assistance Programs." Low-income families should look into these programs if their children need long-term supplies of name brand medicines. Some programs offer a discount card for you to use at a traditional pharmacy, while others mail you the medicines once you're enrolled in the program. Contact information for some of the larger companies' programs as well as other prescription assistance information sources are listed at the end of this chapter.

Mental Health

Unfortunately, many insurance plans "carve out" mental health for separate coverage, or for no coverage at all. This doesn't mean that mental illnesses aren't real or aren't disabling—it's simply a way for the insurance carrier to limit costs, and offer cheaper premiums to the employer that is picking up the tab. What do you do if your child needs help from a mental health professional? Fortunately, insiders know there are ways around the system.

Although serious and rare mental health disorders like schizophrenia or severe obsessive-compulsive disorder really do need to be treated by a psychiatrist, some other problems can probably be handled by other professionals in your community. Your insurance carrier will probably cover therapy for these conditions as long as it is not through a psychiatrist. Some common mental health problems are more likely than others to be well-managed by a nonpsychiatrist.

Attention-Deficit Disorder

This should first be treated through the school, using accommodations and other educational interventions. The next step under most circumstances would be to work with a school or community psychologist for appropriate testing. If your child is unable to keep up and medications need to be considered, many pediatricians will be able to help you with these decisions. Psychiatric care is needed for the most severe cases, or the unusual child who fails to improve with commonly used medications.

Anxiety Disorders

An experienced pediatrician should be able to help with ordinary phobias and fears, or with common school refusal or school-day stomachaches. Some more pervasive anxiety disorders may require formal psychotherapy from a psychologist or counselor; anti-anxiety medications are best prescribed by a psychiatrist or neurologist if needed.

Substance Abuse

Although your pediatrician can discuss these problems with your teen, anything beyond experimentation needs to be taken seriously. If your child is failing school, losing friends, or getting arrested, then you ought to work with a substance abuse center that has a proven track record with teens. This is a good time to spend your own money to get the best therapy available.

Depression

Depression can be a very serious and disabling condition in teens. You should work with your pediatrician initially to distinguish between depression and physical illness in any child who seems especially sad, isolated, or distant; or in any child who complains of chronic unexplained pain. Because research on medical therapy for depression in children is incomplete and there are potentially serious side effects of medicine, ongoing medical therapy for depression is best monitored by a psychiatrist.

Therapy for these conditions may entail not only the expense of the psychiatric visits but also the cost of medicines, which if prescribed by a psychiatrist may not be covered by insurance. Your pediatrician may be willing to "rewrite" prescriptions from your psychiatrist to save you money. In this situation, it's best to work with both your pediatrician and psychiatrist as collaborators, keeping both doctors involved in decisions. You'll benefit from less expensive medications and from the additional expertise of your pediatrician.

In some communities with very limited child psychiatry coverage, more and more pediatricians and neurologists are treating these conditions. Although not all pediatricians are comfortable with this, we do not want our patients to suffer. Treatment by an experienced and well-intentioned pediatrician may be the best you can do if geography or financial concerns make it impossible for you to work with a psychiatrist.

Developmental Concerns

If your child has had a delay in learning speech, motor, or social skills your pediatrician may want to refer her for physical therapy, speech therapy, or occupational therapy. Unfortunately, evaluation and treatment for these issues is another area that your insurance may deem unworthy of coverage. Some insider tips can help.

Ask your doctor to use the most "medical" sounding diagnosis that is honest and correct. For instance, handwriting problems can be diagnosed as "fine motor delay," but that often will lead to rejection of coverage. A better diagnosis that may be appropriate is "hypotonia," which means poor strength. If your child has speech problems because of hearing issues related to recurring ear infections, he is much more likely to qualify for coverage if the medical nature of the problem is stressed in any documentation provided to the insurance company. Speech therapy for hearing loss caused by frequent ear infections will be covered; speech therapy for "developmental speech delay" will not.

Your state or county may have services for the evaluation and treatment of developmental problems. These programs, often called "Early Intervention," may be able to at least partially cover the cost of ongoing therapy. Ask your pediatrician if this sort of program is available for your child.

For kids of school age, your local elementary school may have access to therapists who can work with your child during school hours at no extra expense. Even if your child is not enrolled in a public school, these services may be available to you—ask.

If your request for coverage for therapy has been denied and you work for a large company, you may be able to have someone from your employer's human resources department intervene on your behalf. If the policy is large, the insurance company may provide coverage for you rather than lose a big contract with your employer.

Dental, Ophthalmology, and Other Miscellaneous Noncovered Services

To control costs, many issues are treated as "nonmedical" by insurance carriers. These include many areas where separate coverage is available, but may not have been purchased by your employer. Vision issues, dental coverage, oral surgery, podiatry, and many other areas that are sometimes treated by nonphysicians are often excluded from coverage. Insurance payment is much more likely if you are referred for a "medical" diagnosis.

For instance, medical insurance will cover an ophthalmologist to evaluate and treat crossed eyes, but not for nearsightedness; they'll cover a dental visit for a tooth abscess, but not for routine cleaning and examinations. A tooth that's broken in an accident might fall into a grey zone of coverage, where better documentation may get the bill covered even if you don't have a dental plan. You should not expect your pediatrician to ever document a fraudulent diagnosis to help you get insurance coverage, but for many issues in a grey zone choosing a more "medical" diagnosis will help you with your insurance carrier.

> ☞ **To increase your chances of insurance coverage, use the most "medical" sounding diagnosis. This is especially necessary for developmental, vision, or dental concerns.**

What to Do with a Big Bill

If the bill is from your primary provider or somewhere else where you know the staff, call them first. Be friendly, and remember that your doctor's staff wants to get money from your insurance company as much as you do. They'll often work together with you to solve problems. In any case, even if the staff can't help they're less likely to turn your account over to a collection agency if they know you're trying to resolve an insurance dispute.

Review the bill for errors, which are common. You may discover that you're being billed for things that didn't occur.

Inquire about state-mandated services. Some states have laws that require insurance companies to pay for a certain length of hospital stay, or for certain services related to particular diagnoses. You can find this information though your state insurance commissioner's office. If the laws of your state require certain benefits, that trumps any language in the insurance policy.

If you don't like waiting on hold, the worst time to call an insurance company is during the lunch hour on Mondays, from noon until 2:00 Eastern time. The best times to call are usually Tuesday through Friday mornings.

If the Insurance Company Still Says No: The Appeal Process

When my wife had problems with her thumb, one doctor supplied her with a splint; when that didn't help a second doctor had a new splint custom fabricated. Both splints were rejected because the policy "does not cover the repair or replacement of appliances." After several phone calls and rejections, we sent photographs of the splints to prove that neither one of them was a replacement or repair. That finally got the bills covered.

If your insurance company refuses to cover charges that you feel should legitimately be paid, keep these tips in mind as you work through the appeal process:

- *Stay organized.* Keep records of what was discussed at every phone call, along with whom you spoke to and when. Though some insurance representatives will refuse to give out their names, get extensions, first names, and anything else that you can keep track of so you know exactly who said what. Ask every representative you speak with to fully document all of your calls.
- *Stay cool.* It will never help to yell at anyone. Be calm and reasonable, and you'll be taken more seriously.
- *Stay on top.* If they say they need a duplicate copy of something, send it right away. Don't drop the ball on your side—keep the pressure up, and follow-up with phone calls to make sure they've gotten what they need to process your appeal. You should also stay on top of the information in your own policy, and know exactly what language is used in your policy to exclude coverage. Address their rejection from a position of strength, knowing exactly what your policy says.
- *Stay personal.* If possible, send information to a specific person with whom you've spoken, rather than to the "claims department."
- *Stay persistent.* Don't give up and pay a bill that should legitimately be covered by your insurance plan. Appeal it to the top of the ladder at the insurance company, and if that fails contact your state insurance commissioner's office.

For reductions in coverage based on "usual and customary" figures, a few extra steps may be required. Find out what laws apply in your state by contacting the state insurance commissioner. Your insurance company may be required to provide you with quotes for the cost of these services at local facilities for you to compare, or you may be able to obtain quotes yourself to send to the insurance company so that they can adjust their estimate. Do not accept their "usual and customary" figures without a fight.

If your insurance company has completed their review and continues to deny coverage for which you are entitled, you next step will be to take your grievance to a government authority. Many states have laws that have set up external review boards whose decisions are binding. Contact your state insurance commissioner's office if you need to pursue this type of appeal.

Unfortunately, it can sometimes feel like you have to fight with your insurance company to get claims paid. It seems like it's their job to deny or delay payment, forcing you to struggle through phone trees and paperwork to get the coverage to which you're entitled. Keep in mind that your doctor has to go through the same hoops to get paid! In any case, it never helps to lose your cool, or to give up too easily. Avoid hassles by keeping in mind the tips in this chapter, and if coverage isn't forthcoming begin the careful and deliberate process of appeal. It takes time, but it's your money.

PATIENT ASSISTANCE PROGRAMS

To help defray the high cost of prescription drugs, many manufacturers sponsor assistance programs for families that need help. If you don't know who makes your child's medicine, look at the label or ask your pharmacist. For manufacturers not listed below, ask your pharmacist for more information or use www.google.com to search for the phrase "Patient Assistance Program" + the name of the pharmaceutical company. To qualify for these programs you must lack other prescription drug coverage and meet low-income requirements.

Abbott	800-222-6885
Astra Zeneca	800-424-3727
Aventis	800-221-4025
Bristol-Myers Squibb	800-736-0003
Glaxo Smith Kline	888-825-5249
Lilly	800-545-6962
Merck	800-727-5400
Novartis	800-277-2254
Pfizer	800-707-8990
Roche	800-285-4484
Schering	800-656-9485
Wyeth	800-568-9938

ADDITIONAL INFORMATION

http://www.needymeds.com

Provides information about free and discounted medication programs, with an alphabetical listing of medications and the contact information to seek coverage.

http://www.pparx.org

This clearinghouse site is run by a collaboration of major drug manufacturers to provide prescription assistance to low-income families. There's an online "wizard" that can walk you through the application process for prescription assistance for each of your medications.

15

THE MEDICAL MALPRACTICE CRISIS AND YOUR CHILDREN

Any discussion of the system of medical malpractice liability and litigation inevitably includes the word "crisis." Though there is disagreement on how to fix it, there seems to be universal acceptance of the idea that what we have now isn't working. However, the complaints voiced by doctors and patients are focusing on the wrong issues. The problem isn't just that doctors are paying too much for malpractice insurance, though this is undoubtedly true. Nor is the main issue that many doctors are practicing defensive medicine to avoid lawsuits. To me, the most disappointing failure of the American system of medical malpractice litigation is that it is not actually accomplishing what it is supposed to do. It is not protecting patients from mistakes, it is not fairly reimbursing individuals who are harmed because of medical errors, and it is not helping anyone prevent more medical errors from occurring. In this chapter, I'll expose the failures of the medical malpractice system: it costs too much, and it just doesn't work.

MALPRACTICE LITIGATION: IT COSTS TOO MUCH

Almost all physicians are forced to carry malpractice insurance. In most states, physicians are forbidden from "going bare." We cannot practice medicine unless we carry malpractice insurance. The amount and type that we must carry is dictated by state law, third party payers, and hospitals. Depending on the state and field of practice, malpractice insurance for a single physician can run from $10,000 to $400,000 per year. Though pediatricians are not a common target of lawsuits, when there is a judgment against us the awards tend to be quite high. Pediatricians also have added risk because we're subject to lawsuits for anything that occurs during a patient's entire childhood. If an adult suffers an injury because of a medical error, the lawsuit must be filed within two years in most states. This "statute of limitations" doesn't apply in pediatrics, where lawsuits can be brought for any action that occurs to a child until they reach age twenty. Despite how infrequently we actually get sued, pediatricians still pay substantially for their malpractice coverage.

Why are premiums so high? There's no single answer, and there is heated disagreement about which of these factors is the most important:

- Jury awards are very high, and getting higher. (This isn't necessarily true; in some states that have capped jury awards there has not been a corresponding decrease in insurance rates.)
- Doctors have failed to weed out the "bad apples"—the handful of doctors who make most of the mistakes.
- Insurance companies have had less income from their other investments, and have had to squeeze more dollars out of premiums than in the past.
- Because of consolidation and decreased competition among malpractice carriers, the insurance companies have been able to increase rates without physicians being able to shop for a less expensive carrier.

Additional costs are incurred by added overhead to prevent and defend lawsuits. For instance, my practice's insurance carrier has recently insisted that we contact every patient that we've suggested should see a specialist to ensure that they really went. These calls should be repeated and documented, and once the specialist visit is completed, we're expected to badger the specialist for proof in writing that the visit took place. Furthermore, our insurance company thinks that if the specialist ordered any sort of tests or further follow-up, we need to continue to contact the family to ensure that everything that was suggested was actually done. There is extra cost to my practice for employees to take care of all of this. Of course the insurance company isn't offering to pay for it, or cut my malpractice premiums—they just expect us to do it and absorb the cost ourselves.

There is an even more insidious cost, beyond the direct costs of insurance and the indirect costs of employee time to keep up with added overhead. The most serious and regrettable consequence of a fear of lawsuits is the effect this is having on the relationship between physicians and their patients.

- Doctors have become very reluctant to phone in prescriptions. We're fearful that a telephone diagnosis might be wrong, and we'll get sued. Though we really would sometimes like to do you a favor and help you over the phone, we are reluctant to take on any extra risk of an imperfect diagnosis.
- We're going to spend more time documenting things in the chart, which means less time talking with you. Our charts have to be complete to defend us against lawsuits. We spend extra time charting, and see extra patients to

cover the costs of malpractice fears. So there's less time to actually interact with our patients. The practice of medicine would be better if doctors had more time to concentrate on patients rather than charts.

- Doctors are reluctant to use e-mail or give meaningful telephone advice. Again, anything that increases our risk is going to be avoided. Besides, physicians are understandably reluctant to assume extra risk for telephone calls that we traditionally do for free. Whenever we have to make a decision without actually seeing the patient we are more likely to overlook something and make a mistake. Also, a brief typed answer may not contain all of the advice we would have said in person—especially for doctors who type slowly. Yet those few typed words are entirely admissible in court.
- Doctors are reluctant to criticize other doctors. In part, this is from a spirit of collegiality among our profession; but we really don't want to be dragged into any sort of lawsuit, as a defendant or a witness. It certainly makes sense not to encourage frivolous lawsuits, but the fearfulness of litigation has led to a regrettable hesitancy among doctors to engage in honest criticism and discussion of the actions of other doctors. There may well be more than one way to do something correctly, and patients would be better served if their pediatrician would be more open about the decisions being made by other doctors.
- Doctors are more likely to practice "defensive medicine." That is, we're more likely to order tests, refer to specialists, and send patients to the emergency room. This dramatically increases the amount of money spent on medical care, and subjects many patients to unnecessary and painful procedures that are unlikely to help. We can't allow any chance of a mistake or any chance of a missed diagnosis. In an effort to leave no stone unturned, we're making an expensive and painful mess.

To some degree, there is another side to these examples. Phoned-in medicines are in fact more likely to be incorrect than prescriptions presented in writing, and better documented charts are more medically helpful for the doctor to review later. But clearly the relationship of patient to doctor is changing, in part because of this fear of litigation. Rather than a friendly partnership, the relationship between a family and their pediatrician now has an element of fear and defensiveness that colors every interaction.

MALPRACTICE LITIGATION: IT DOESN'T WORK

Malpractice attorneys contend that civil litigation is a necessary element to protect patients. To an extent they are correct. I would certainly agree that patients harmed by medical errors should be compensated, and that physicians and hospitals who are the cause of mistakes should bear the burden of compensation for people who suffer as a result of those mistakes—a simple application of the universally accepted principle "you break it, you buy it." By encouraging medical systems to identify and fix sources of medical errors, a consequence of malpractice litigation should be safer medical care for all.

However, the malpractice system as it exists now fails to accomplish these worthwhile goals.

Malpractice lawsuits don't fairly compensate most victims of malpractice. Most patients harmed by medical malpractice do not sue their doctor. In fact, less than 3 percent of people who suffer medical injury as a result of an error get any compensation at all. As to the awards given to people who prevail in a lawsuit or settlement, less than half of the money actually goes to the victims. Even this is often delayed by years as the case drags through the legal system.

Physicians who have not been sued still bear most of the costs of malpractice litigation. Only about one in three pediatricians are sued during their careers; a tiny minority gets sued more than five times. Yet the cost of malpractice coverage has skyrocketed for all pediatricians, including those of us who are practicing the most careful medicine.

Sources of errors are not being identified and fixed. In part because of the fear of lawsuits, physicians are reluctant to face the cause of errors head on. We'd rather not have systems in place to look for errors because this will give ammunition to lawyers looking for lucrative lawsuits.

Why Doesn't It Work?

As we've seen, the current system of medical malpractice has huge costs. It is too expensive, and it has reduced the ability of doctors to be helpful to families. At the same time, it is not fairly compensating victims, it is not punishing the perpetrators of errors, and it is not protecting your family from medical errors. Why doesn't the system work? Though again many honest people disagree about the problems facing our litigation system, many root problems are easy to identify.

It is clear that the malpractice litigation process is too cumbersome, expensive, and lengthy. It cannot be navigated without lawyers, and because lawyers work on contingency they will only want to represent a "slam-dunk" winnable case. Once representation is hired, it may take years for a monetary award or settlement to reach the injured party. Many patients who deserve compensation following a harmful error are reluctant to begin this overwhelming and time consuming process.

In addition, lawsuits are often filed against doctors who have not made mistakes. For instance, doctors who are poor communicators—or who lack warm relationships with their patients—are far more likely to get sued. Though being able to get along with your patients is a good skill for any doctor to have, a lack of this relationship shouldn't be the main reason to be served with a lawsuit. Apart from lawsuits filed for reasons of personality over practice, other lawsuits are filed solely because of bad outcomes rather than bad decisions. Not every bad outcome is the result of a medical error. Some things are out of a physician's control; even the best medicine cannot adequately treat some of the worst diseases. Yet in our society, perfection is expected, and unfortunate circumstances attract lawsuits when no one is to blame. Only genuine medical errors are meant to be compensated by malpractice awards, yet the system now allows and even encourages lawsuits for the wrong reasons.

One of the most common reasons for obstetricians to be sued is that they delivered a baby who later developed evidence of brain problems, like cerebral palsy (CP). Although in the past it was believed that CP was often caused by damage that occurred to the brain during birth (presumably because the baby wasn't delivered correctly), it is now well established that most children with CP suffered their injury long before delivery, and that this injury could not have been prevented by any doctor despite the best modern technology. Nonetheless, because CP can be such a sad and devastating problem it continues to drive many lucrative lawsuits against obstetricians.

The current adversarial system may not be the best way to arrive at a fair decision. Each side in a lawsuit has its own expert witnesses to testify to their own point of view, with a judge and jury expected to decide who is right. But medical decisions are complex, and it may be difficult for persons outside of the medical field to make informed decisions without overly relying on these hired gun "experts." Though some states have passed laws to curtail the use of "professional" expert witnesses testifying for whoever has the most money, too often the outcome is decided by the quality and presentation of the experts rather than the impartial facts of the case. Meanwhile, the expert witnesses get paid hundreds of dollars an hour or more, attracting people motivated by greed rather than a desire to offer truthful and unbiased testimony.

WHAT SHOULD BE DONE?

Tort Reform

Several solutions for so-called "tort reform" are being hotly debated and enacted in some states.

Caps on Noneconomic Damages

How much is an injury worth? "Actual damages" refers to time missed from work, the expense of medical bills, and other easily measured items. But malpractice awards may include further damages, for "pain and suffering" or "punitive damages" to further punish the person who committed the mistake. In many states, efforts are underway to put a cap on these "noneconomic" damages, limiting them to less than $500,000 to $1,000,000. The idea is that if huge, "jackpot" jury awards are eliminated, fewer lawsuits will be filed. Based on data from states that have passed these caps, it is not yet clear that caps will consistently lead to a dramatic decrease in malpractice insurance rates.

"Loser Pays"

To help weed out frivolous lawsuits, under a "loser pays" system the party that loses the lawsuit has to pay the legal fees of the other side, regardless of or in addition to any sort of award. Though this has a certain appeal, from a practical point of view it is difficult to know if this sort of system would deter many unjustified lawsuits. It would certainly discourage less wealthy people from bringing any case to court for fear of bankruptcy. An opposing side could deliberately run up litigation costs just to make the other side more fearful of their potential losses if they lose the case.

Impartial Experts

Under current law, all "expert witnesses" are hired by one side or another. Both the plaintiff and the defense can bring in their own hired experts, who can be expected to have a certain slant to their testimony as they work to help their own side prevail. In some jurisdictions, the courts themselves can bring in experts from the community that have no allegiance to either side in the dispute. Court-appointed experts can freely give testimony based on their independent opinions of the merits of the case.

Pretrial Screening

If required, pretrial screening by an independent review board can determine if there is any merit to a case before it heads to court. The review board should consist of members of both the medical and lay communities, as boards stocked only by doctors might be overly sympathetic to physicians.

Beyond Tort Reform

Though the above measures may help, insiders know there are other steps that need to be taken. Most importantly, doctors need to stop defending each other, and focus on defending their patients. Every doctor knows a handful of practicing physician colleagues that are lousy physicians—doctors that we would never send our own family members to see. Yet we are very reluctant to identify such practitioners. Most state medical boards are staffed entirely by physicians reluctant to take any meaningful action against a doctor's license, even after repeated mistakes are made. A first step toward improving the medical malpractice landscape is for physicians to have high expectations of each other, and to be willing to identify and kick out the physicians who are doing a lousy job.

Doctors also need to be more honest with patients about the expectations of therapy and treatment, and to honestly disclose mistakes when they do occur. The next chapter explores more about medical errors and what you can do to prevent them from affecting your family.

The Best Solution

Medical malpractice litigation ought to have two goals: (1) there should be adequate compensation for people injured as the result of medical errors, and (2) the system should encourage doctors and hospitals to address the specific causes of errors so that fewer people are injured in the first place. The best way to meet these goals may be to replace the entire medical malpractice liability system with a mandatory system of no-fault compensation for medical errors, similar to the workman's compensation program for occupational injuries. Under such a system, an injured party would not have to fight with their doctor or hospital; they would only need to prove to an impartial administrator that they were injured, and that the injury was a result of a medical decision or procedure. Any valid claim would receive appropriate compensation from a central fund, which would be supported by relatively small premiums from physicians and hospitals. Because no "blame" is assigned, health care providers would be much more willing to report and study the causes of errors, improving patient safety. Risk management strategies would evolve with a goal of actually preventing errors, and not just preventing blame.

For now, though, such an ideal system does not seem likely to evolve. Too many people are benefiting from the current system—lawyers, insurance companies, and legislators—for any dramatic changes to occur in the near future. Though you should be aware of how a fear of malpractice litigation is affecting the relationship between your family and your pediatrician, you cannot depend on litigation fears to drive any meaningful effort to decrease medical errors. In the next chapter, I'll tell you exactly how a pediatric insider suggests you take your own steps toward preventing medical errors from harming your child.

> **The current medical malpractice system will not protect you from medical errors, poorly run hospitals, or lousy doctors.**

16

Everyone Makes Mistakes

In 1999, the Institute of Medicine released *To Err is Human*, a groundbreaking review of medical errors occurring in hospitals in the United States. A shocking statistic was published: each year, medical errors directly cause 44,000 to 98,000 deaths. The authors compared this to one jumbo jet crashing each and every day.

Although the exact number of deaths is debatable, the report and other reviews of both inpatient and outpatient medical errors have shown that a large number of preventable errors continues to plague the medical system, resulting in a tremendous amount of pain, worry, and loss of life. Although many physicians and health administrators are working diligently to reduce this problem, there are things that every family should do to prevent a medical error from harming their child. In this chapter we'll look at an insider's picture of why medical errors occur, and how families can try to steer out of their way.

What kind of mistakes are we talking about?

- Wrong medicines
- Wrong doses
- Wrong diagnoses
- Wrong tests ordered
- Wrong results reported
- And many more. If you can imagine it happening, it has happened, and probably more than once.

Some case examples:

- A pediatrician orders a wrong vaccine on a child. After it is administered, the nurse realizes that the vaccine is not usually given at that age; after conferring with other nurses, she speaks with the doctor and confirms that the mistake was made. Fortunately, the extra unneeded dose is unlikely to harm the baby, but the parents are so upset they refuse to allow the correct vaccine to be given. The family leaves the practice.

- A father from Venezuela is given a prescription to control his son's heart condition. A few days later the child is brought to the hospital unconscious, with a dangerously low blood pressure. It is discovered that his father reading the medicine label interpreted the instructions "give 1 tablet once a day" to mean give the tablet eleven times a day. "Once" means eleven in Spanish. The child recovers after a day in the intensive care unit.
- A child is brought to the pediatrician for an itchy rash. The family gives the medicine as instructed − 4 ounces at bedtime—but rather than spread it on the child's skin, they give the medicine orally. The child has several seizures and needs aggressive therapy in the intensive care unit. Years later, his troubles in school are thought to be a result of this incident.

WHY DO MISTAKES OCCUR?

Understanding the circumstances that contribute to errors is the first step in avoiding them. Most medical errors do not occur as the fault of single individual, but as the result of a system that is not designed to prevent errors in a systematic way.

Medicine supports a culture that does not question or second guess doctors. Doctors, of course, are human. We make mistakes. Unfortunately nurses and support people are reluctant to question a doctor's orders even when they suspect something is wrong.

Medical systems do not encourage the reporting and tracking of errors. This is at least partially because of a fear of litigation. In most states, if a medical error is carefully investigated and steps are made to prevent a recurrence, this will make it easier for the plaintiff's attorneys to win their lawsuit.

Medical care is disjointed. Patients see several doctors, and get labs and x-rays from a variety of places. They do not necessarily visit the same pharmacy for every prescription, and may take a variety of potent over-the-counter medicines.

Doctors sometimes practice outside of their area of expertise. In some communities or with some insurance plans, access to specialists is difficult. Some doctors feel forced to use unfamiliar medicines to treat unfamiliar conditions. This is especially a problem with child psychiatry. There are far too few well-qualified child psychiatrists, and many insurance plans do not cover their care. Very, very few psychiatric medicines are approved for use in children, and general community pediatricians have limited training in dealing with serious psychiatric problems. There is a huge potential for error when poorly trained physicians use poorly studied medicines.

Patients have no reliable way to tell how many mistakes are occurring. A savvy medical shopper would like to choose a hospital and a doctor's office where medical mistakes are uncommon, but this information is difficult to obtain. You might be able to find out how many lawsuits are pending or settled against a doctor, but that may not accurately reflect how many errors are occurring in that office. Most medical mistakes do not result in a lawsuit, and many lawsuits are filed even when no mistake has occurred.

Bad doctors and nurses are not identified and sanctioned. Although everyone makes mistakes, it is certainly true that some health care professionals are more sloppy and prone to mistakes than others. Every doctor knows several colleagues they would never allow to treat their own family, yet in most states very few doctors or nurses have their license suspended because of repeated mistakes.

Doctors and nurses give many instructions to patients and each other orally. Verbal information is easily misunderstood and is not always remembered correctly. Nurses should repeat back all verbal instructions, and should not accept verbal orders for any dangerous procedure or medicine. Verbal communication can also lead to errors when doctors give instructions to families. For complex problems or complex patients, many new instructions are given at every visit. Few of these are written down, and I suspect that few of them are remembered correctly.

Doctors do not communicate well between themselves. Complex patients often see several different doctors for their problems, and each doctor may prescribe different treatments. Although most specialists write letters to the primary care giver, these may take weeks to arrive, and are not always available for easy review at the next visit.

WHAT SHOULD FAMILIES DO?

These problems are deeply rooted in medical culture and training, and are unlikely to go away anytime soon. However, there is hope. Diligent physicians, nurses, hospital administrators, and academics are working on many of these issues, with considerable success in at least a few centers. But it will take years to change the culture of medicine to one that recognizes human errors will always occur. In the meantime, what can your family do to avoid a medical mistake?

Be an active and inquisitive member of your child's health care team. Ask questions and expect answers. If you don't know what's going on you're less likely to be able to spot a problem. Ask why tests and procedures are being done, and ask why medications are being prescribed. Research your child's issues through reliable sources (see Chapter 12).

Insist on clear communication. When the visit is complete, you should know the exact diagnosis and plan, including all care instructions, medicines, and doses. If you don't understand instructions, ask the doctor to repeat them and write them down. Many medical words are new to parents; do not be shy about asking the physician to write terms down so you can do your own research later. If your child is hospitalized, make sure you know the exact plan for treatment and follow-up when you are sent home.

Choose a doctor who is humble and listens. A doctor who is humble doesn't mind when others help her spot mistakes. A doctor who listens to her patients and her staff has much more than her own eyes and ears to catch problems. Everyone involved in the care of a child—from the child herself to the parents, nurses, receptionists, and doctor—has a responsibility to be vigilant and aware that human errors can occur. But if the doctor doesn't listen to anyone but herself, the errors will not be fixed. Your doctor should be confident, but not cocky.

Choose an office with a happy staff. Happy staff are not rushed or pressured. They are more comfortable speaking up and are less afraid to point out a mistake. Unhappy staff may well let an error go by without speaking up.

> ☞ **The best way to prevent errors is to insist on clear, open, and complete communication between families and physicians.**

Office recordkeeping should be clear. Many offices now use a computerized medical record. Although these do not automatically prevent all medical errors, a well-run computerized record can be a tremendous help. Whether electronic or traditional, the medical record should be clear, organized, and legible. If your doctor's office is always losing paper and can't put their hands on your information right away, errors are far more prone to occur.

Keep your own clean records of medical information, and share this with all of the doctors involved in your child's care. You should know all of your child's medicines and doses, all allergies, and any important past medical problems. If you have trouble keeping track of this, write it down. Although you should expect your own physician to know all of this from the child's chart, keep your own records to be sure. If you visit an outside medical facility (such as an emergency room), bring all of the records from that visit to your doctor. These records should include the notes from the doctor who saw you, plus lab and x-ray results.

Be certain that all treating physicians know every medicine your child takes. If your child sees more than one doctor who is prescribing medications, the best way to ensure that all of his doctors know all of his medicines is to bring all of them with you to appointments. Bringing a brown lunch bag of medicines with you is a simple step that can ensure every doctor knows what medicines are being taken. Don't forget to tell every doctor about over-the-counter products and herbal supplements, too.

Know your child's medication allergies in detail. Know what happened when your child took what drug. There may be circumstances where a presumed allergy might be "low-risk," and trying the medicine again might be the best decision. You should know not only the names of any medicine that has led to a reaction, but the exact detailed history of any reaction that has occurred.

You should be able to read every handwritten prescription. Some of the letters may be in code, but you should be able to read the words and numbers. Double check every medicine when you pick it up from the pharmacy—is it what you expected?

Learn how to administer your child's medicines. Liquids need to be measured; inhaled medicines sometimes need special devices and instructions. Ask your doctor or pharmacist how to give all medicines in the best way.

> ☞ **If you can't read a prescription, neither can the pharmacist.**

Follow up on any tests. Ask when to expect results of any test or x-ray, and call your doctor if you haven't heard the results in a reasonable amount of time. Don't assume that no news is good news. Sometimes a fax is misplaced or results are not sent to your doctor. You're in the best position to ensure that all results are reviewed and interpreted.

If your child needs surgery, choose a surgeon who is experienced and a site where the procedure is done often. There is a better chance of success when both the surgeon and the facility have done plenty of the procedures. You don't want to be the "cool case of the day"—you'd rather be one of hundreds or thousands of identical procedures done successfully over the course of many years.

Insist that health care workers wash their hands. Infections that are caught at a medical visit are a significant health problem, and so-called "nosocomial infections" are a leading cause of death among very ill patients in intensive care units. Many of the germs that lurk at health care facilities are particularly virulent and hard to treat, and can be an especially vexing problem when

> ☞ **The single best way to prevent the spread of disease-causing microorganisms is thorough hand washing with soap and water or a hand sanitizing solution.**

they strike a child who is already ill. Your best protection is frequent and thorough hand washing by yourself, your child, and all health care providers. If you haven't seen the doctors or nurses wash or sanitize their hands, speak up.

If you have trouble with English, be positive that everything said is understood. Ideally, choose a physician who speaks your native language well. A mature interpreter is a second best solution. Don't rely on a bilingual child to act as an interpreter in a medical encounter; kids may lack the maturity to understand medical questions or relay information accurately.

Speak up. If you think you've spotted a problem, bring it up with your doctor. If you've just got a question, bring that up too. You have a responsibility as a parent to speak up and help protect your child if something is not going right.

You can't expect your physician or medical office to never make a mistake. In fact, a historic refusal to admit mistakes has contributed to a medical culture that is not geared toward preventing errors. But by choosing a medical office that is well run and insisting on clear communication between doctors, nurses, and patients, you can reduce the risk that a medical error will harm your child.

Appendix: Fun with Medical Statistics

The best way to understand the effectiveness of medical interventions or the accuracy of tests is to review the scientific studies of their performance. Exactly how well does this new medicine work? How reliable is the result of that study? Statements like "this new drug is better than the old one" or "this test result means you probably don't have cancer" may be all that some patients need to know, but other patients want a better understanding of the details. What do doctors know, and how sure are we about the results of the studies that we quote and rely on every day?

I'll tell you right upfront: these details are going to be a little difficult to follow. This is only for those of you who really want to know the fundamental truths behind medical tests. If you understand this section, you'll have a better handle on medical statistics than most practicing physicians. A thorough review of medical statistics is far beyond the scope of this book. But for those of you who are curious, this appendix will review some of the statements from earlier chapters, explaining in more detail the mathematics and statistics that are the foundation of the science of medicine.

If There Is No Statistical Difference between Two Results, There Is No Difference at All

This quote from Chapter 10 refers to the inexact nature of numerical results. When a study determines, say, how many days of fever a child with an ear infection is likely to have, the most commonly reported result in the newspaper is usually the average result—let's say, 3.0 days. But in a medical journal, this result is usually expressed as a "confidence interval," or a range. The same result might appear alternatively as "3.0 ± .5 days" or "2.5–3.5 days." The table will probably also give a numeric qualifier to the result, usually a percentage close to 100 percent. This percentage expresses the statistical confidence that the experimentally measured result reflects the true result. A result expressed as "3.0 ± .5 days, 95 percent confidence interval" means that the study determined with 95 percent confidence that the true length of fever is between 2.5 and 3.5 days.

If two items are being compared, look to see if the confidence intervals overlap. Let's say the patients in group A took only placebo, and their average length of fever was "3.0 ± .5 days." The kids in group B, who took the new antibiotic "Payolacillin," had a fever for "2.6 ± .5 days." Though the newspaper account will say that the period of fever was shorter with the new drug, by looking more closely at the results we see that the two confidence intervals overlap. The average fever for one group was anywhere from 2.5–3.5 days, and in the other group it was 2.1–3.1 days—which means that in fact the two groups could really have had fever for the same number of days! The numbers 2.5–3.1 are in both intervals, so there is *no statistical difference* between the groups.

The newspaper account for this result should read: "A new study showed that the drug Payolacillin did not help shorten the days of fever," or even more accurately, "A new study failed to show that Payolacillin was better than placebo." Confidence intervals that overlap between the two results being compared means that the study failed to prove that there was any difference.

Studies that have wide intervals—like "3.0 ± 2.0 days"—have one of two problems. Either they had too few subjects, or there was a tremendous amount of variability in the number of days of fever among the study participants. In either case, the average value of 3.0 can't be trusted—the true value could be anywhere from 1 to 5 days.

Another way of expressing the same idea is through reporting a "*p* value." The *p* value of a result is the statistical probability that the result occurred by chance alone. The more "reliable" the result is—that is, the more data that statistically shows the result to be more likely to be true—the lower the *p* value. In medicine, a *p* value of .05 is considered to be a cutoff below which a result is considered to be meaningful. Often, a study will express a result along with a *p* value to reinforce that the author's statistical analysis shows the result to be valid. A meaningful result includes a notation that "$p < .05$," or an exact value like "$p = .006$." Note that any result with a *p* value less than .05 is considered to have statistically demonstrated the result; a smaller *p* value doesn't count extra. Do not be more impressed with a $p = .001$ than a $p = .01$; both have proven their point, statistically speaking. Sometimes poorly designed studies trumpet their tiny *p* values in the hope that this will obscure other design shortcomings. Don't be fooled.

THE MORE TESTS YOU DO, THE MORE THE CHANCE THAT ONE WILL BE ABNORMAL, EVEN IF NOTHING IS WRONG

Chapter 13 included this observation, and the math to prove it is not too difficult. Let's say a single test has an accuracy of 95 percent. That is, 95 percent of the time, the result of the test is correct.

If you do this single test once, you'll get an accurate result 95 percent of the time. But let's say you do two tests, each of which has 95 percent accuracy. What's the chance that *both* of them are correct?

In probability, to determine if two events both occur you multiply their chances together. In this case, with two tests, the chance of them both being correct is .95 × .95 = .90. (Results in the appendix are rounded to two decimal places.) By doing two tests, the chance that at least one of them is wrong is already 10 percent.

A general formula for determining the chance that all results of a series of tests are correct is: $C = a^n$, where C is the chance of all correct answers, a is the accuracy of any single test, and n is the number of tests done.

Using 95 percent accuracy, for ten tests your chance of them all being correct is 60 percent; for thirty tests the chance of all correct tests is only 21 percent. Even using 99 percent accuracy, if thirty tests are done you'd expect all accurate results only 74 percent of the time. And if you add up the components of the blood tests that are done routinely, you'll quickly get past thirty individual tests.

Even when tests are accurate, if you do enough of them you're bound to end up with some incorrect results.

IF THE DISEASE IS VERY UNLIKELY, A POSITIVE TEST RESULT IS PROBABLY WRONG

The quote from Chapter 13 should more formally be stated: as the probability of a true positive result becomes lower, it becomes more and more likely that any positive result is actually false. The opposite statement is also equally true: if a disease is very *likely*, than a *negative* test result is probably wrong. This is a consequence of computations using Bayes' Theorem, which is the key computation in figuring out the true likelihood of disease given the results of a test.

Tests have their own inherent characteristics that tell you how accurate they are. These characteristics answer the questions "Among a group of people who have a condition, how many of them will have a positive test?" (the sensitivity) AND "Among a group of people who do *not* have a condition, how many of them will have a negative test?" (the specificity).

The sensitivity and specificity of a test are statistical terms used in medicine and many other areas of science and technology. They are inherent to the test itself, assuming that the test is performed correctly and consistently.

But in fact what you *really* want to know are those questions asked the other way around: "If my child has a positive test, what is the chance he really has the disease?" (the positive predictive value) or "If my child has a negative test, what is the chance that he truly doesn't have the disease?" (The negative predictive value). Unlike the sensitivity and specificity, these positive and negative predictive values are not inherent to the test itself, but rely also on the prevalence of the disease. The positive predictive value of a test is always greater if the disease is more common; conversely, the negative predictive value of a test is always lower if a disease is rare.

To know your child's chance of truly having a condition based on the result of the test, you need to know not only the characteristics and accuracy of the test itself, but also the chance that he really has the disease that's being tested, or the "pretest probability." That is, what's the chance that he has the condition, even before the test is done? Among children with your child's characteristics and history and physical exam, how many of them have the illness that's detected by the test?

The chance of a child truly having disease, or the posttest probability, is calculated using Bayes' Theorem. For a positive test result, the posttest probability = pretest probability ∗ sensitivity/[pretest probability ∗ sensitivity + (1 − pretest probability) ∗ (1 − specificity)].

What's important to remember isn't the formula, it's that the chance of your child truly having a disease depends not only on the accuracy (a loose way of saying "the sensitivity and specificity") of the test, but also the pretest probability. If the pretest probability is low, unless the test is very accurate a positive test will not prove that the child has disease. It will more likely be wrong.

Some computed examples, in tabular form, are presented below. For brevity I'm presenting only examples of positive tests, but a similar table could be created to reinforce the converse point, that is, if the disease is very likely, a negative test still doesn't prove that the child doesn't have the disease.

Sensitivity	Specificity	Pretest probability (%)	Posttest probability (%)
.95	.95	1	16
.95	.95	10	68
.95	.95	50	95
.80	.80	10	31
.80	.80	20	50

Note: Examples of tests, including their characteristic sensitivities and specificities. In each row, a pretest probability is shown along with the corresponding posttest probability if the test were positive.

As the table shows, even for an excellent test (both sensitivity and specificity are 95 percent), if the pretest probability is low (1 percent) the computed posttest probability is still well below 50 percent—meaning that the positive test result was wrong! Once the pretest probability climbs to 10 percent, most of the time the positive results are correct, but still 32 percent of the time the child doesn't truly have the disease. The lower part of the table shows a test with 80 percent sensitivity and specificity—that's quite typical of many ordinary tests that doctors use. If the doctor estimated that there was a 1 in 5 chance of your child having the disease (a pretest probability of 20 percent), then even with a positive test result the chance of truly having disease is only 50 percent. The doctor could have just flipped a coin to get the same information!

The exact sensitivities and specificities are often only estimated for many of the tests that doctors order, and it is doubtful that many pediatricians go through this formal calculation. But both you and your pediatrician should understand that in a case where the pretest probability of disease is either very high or very low, unless a test is nearly perfect its result cannot be relied upon to really prove or disprove a disease. In other words: if you really doubt a diagnosis is possible, don't do the test; likewise, if you're sure that a diagnosis has already been made, don't do the test. Only the most super-accurate tests should be performed if the pretest probabilities are either very high or very low, or an unexpected result is more likely to be an error than the truth.

INDEX

About the Author

ROY BENAROCH, M.D. is Clinical Assistant Professor of Pediatrics at Emory University, and a Pediatrician with a practice in Roswell, Georgia. The father of three children, "Dr. Roy" completed an undergraduate degree in Biomedical Engineering at Tulane University and completed medical school and his residency at Emory University.

About the Series Editor

JULIE SILVER, M.D., is Assistant Professor, Harvard Medical School, Department of Physical Medicine and Rehabilitation, and a Clinical Associate in Physiatry at Brigham & Women's Hospital and Massachusetts General Hospital. She is also Medical Director at Spaulding Outpatient Center as well as Attending Physician at Spaulding Rehabilitation Hospital. Silver has authored, edited, or co-edited twelve books in addition to journal articles, and columns for *Special Living and Unique Opportunities.* Silver is also editor of the newsletter for the International Rehabilitation Center for Polio. Her awards include the American Medical Writers Association Solimene Award for Excellence in Medical Writing. Silver is the founder and director of an annual seminar facilitated by the Harvard Medical School Department of Continuing Education, "Publishing Books, Memoirs and Other Creative Non-Fiction."